Early Magnetism In Its Higher Relations To Humanity: As Veiled In The Poets And The Prophets

Thomas South

EARLY MAGNETISM

IN ITS

HIGHER RELATIONS TO HUMANITY,

AS

VEILED IN THE POETS AND THE PROPHETS.

BY

ΘΥΟΣ ΜΑΘΟΣ.

That is the great inscrutable mystery, open before all
Eyes, encompassing all space, but by no one is seen.
SCHILLER.

"Enquire I pray thee of the former age, and prepare thyself to the search of
their fathers."—JOB VIII. 8.

LONDON:

H. BAILLIERE, PUBLISHER,

219, REGENT STREET,

FOREIGN BOOKSELLER TO THE ROYAL COLLEGE OF SURGEONS AND THE
ROYAL MEDICO-CHIRURGICAL SOCIETY.

PARIS: J. B. BAILLIERE, LIBRAIRE DE L'ACADEMIE ROYALE DE
MEDECINE, RUE DE L'ECOLE DE MEDECINE.

MDCCCXLVI.

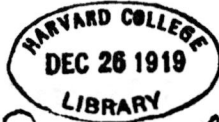

LONDON:
Printed by Schulze and Co., 13, Poland Street.

PREFACE.

THE motive which has drawn forth this small
work is, it is believed, a very ordinary one, that
of offering back again for the service of Truth,
knowledge which has been pleasurably and
gratefully gathered. In the present negative and
transitional state of the Scientific World general
approval is little hoped for ; it is therefore only
to the enlightened believing few, whose thought-
ful experience has enabled them to appreciate
the great magnetical revelation of the true Light
of Nature, that the Author looks for encourage-
ment to cheer his spirit, hesitating to pass on
from this Introduction to a fuller and more open
exposition of truths, bearing, as he conceives,
on the highest and best interests of the Human
Race.

A translation of the few Latin quotations has been proposed for the general reader. But as they were appealed to and adduced by the Author not only to sanction, but to energize and give higher tone to his ideas, would not his translating them be again to lose in literal dulness what he sought to gain in classical point and application? In case, however, they should prove troublesome to any reader, disinclined to pass them over, prose translations are given in notes appended to the end. Conscious want of language to convey such yet unfamiliar conceptions, in utterance equal and responsive to the sense deep and newly stirred that gave them birth, was the occasion of introducing them.

SELECT CATALOGUE

OF

WORKS ON MESMERISM,

&c. &c.

LATELY PUBLISHED

BY HIPPOLYTE BAILLIERE,

219, *REGENT STREET.*

J. ALLISON, M.D.

MESMERISM; its Pretentions as a Science physiologically considered. By J. Allison, M.D. 8vo. London, 1844. 1s.

JOHN ELLIOTSON, M.D. Cantab. F.R.S.

NUMEROUS CASES OF SURGICAL OPERATIONS without Pain in the Mesmeric State; with Remarks upon the Opposition of many Members of the Royal Medical and Chirurgical Society and others, to the reception of the inestimable blessings of Mesmerism. By John Elliotson, M.D. 8vo. London, 1843. 2s. 6d.

THE HARVEIAN ORATION, delivered before the Royal College of Physicians, London, June 27, 1846. By John Elliotson, M.D. With an English Version and Notes. 8vo. London, 1846. 2s. 6d.

W. C. ENGLEDUE, M.D.

CEREBRAL PHYSIOLOGY AND MATERIALISM, with the Result of the Application of Animal Magnetism to the Cerebral Organs. An Address delivered to the Phrenological Association in London, June 20, 1842. By W. C. Engledue, M.D. With a Letter from John Elliotson, M.D. 8vo. London, 1842. 1s.

MRS. LAVINIA JONES.

THE CURATIVE POWER of Vital Magnetism, verified by actual Application to numerous Cases of Disease. By Mrs. Lavinia Jones. 18mo. London, 1845. 1s.

SANDBY & KISTE.

MESMERISM; or, Facts against Fallacies. In a Letter to the Rev. George Sandby. By A. Kiste. 18mo. London, 1845. 1s.

HENRY STORER, M.D.

MESMERISM IN DISEASE; a Few Plain Facts, with a Selection of Cases. By Henry Storer, M.D. Second Edition, 12mo. London, 1845. 2s. 6d.

M. TESTE, M.D.

A PRACTICAL MANUAL OF ANIMAL MAGNETISM; containing an Exposition of the Methods employed in producing the Magnetic Phenomena, with its Application to the Treatment and Cure of Diseases. From the second edition. By D. Spillan, M.D. Dedicated, with permission, to John Elliotson, M.D. Cantab. F.R.S. 1 vol. post 8vo. London, 1843. 6s.

TOPHAM & WARD.

ACCOUNT of a Case of Successful Amputation of the Thigh during the Mesmeric State without the knowledge of the Patient. Read to the Royal Medical and Chirurgical Society on the 22nd November, 1842. By W. Topham, Esq. and W. S. Ward, Esq. 8vo. 1842. 1s.

REV. C. H. TOWNSHEND.

FACTS IN MESMERISM, with Reasons for a Dispassionate Inquiry into it. Second edition, with a New Preface and enlarged. 8vo. London, 1844. 9s.

THE ZOIST. A Journal of Mesmerism.

A JOURNAL OF CEREBRAL PHYSIOLOGY AND MESMERISM, and their application to Human Welfare. Published Quarterly. Price of each Number, 2s. 6d.
This Journal contains papers by Drs. Elliotson and Engledue.
Fourteen Numbers have already appeared.
———— Nos. I to XII. in cloth boards, 3 vols. 8vo. 1l. 13s.
Commenced April 1, 1843.

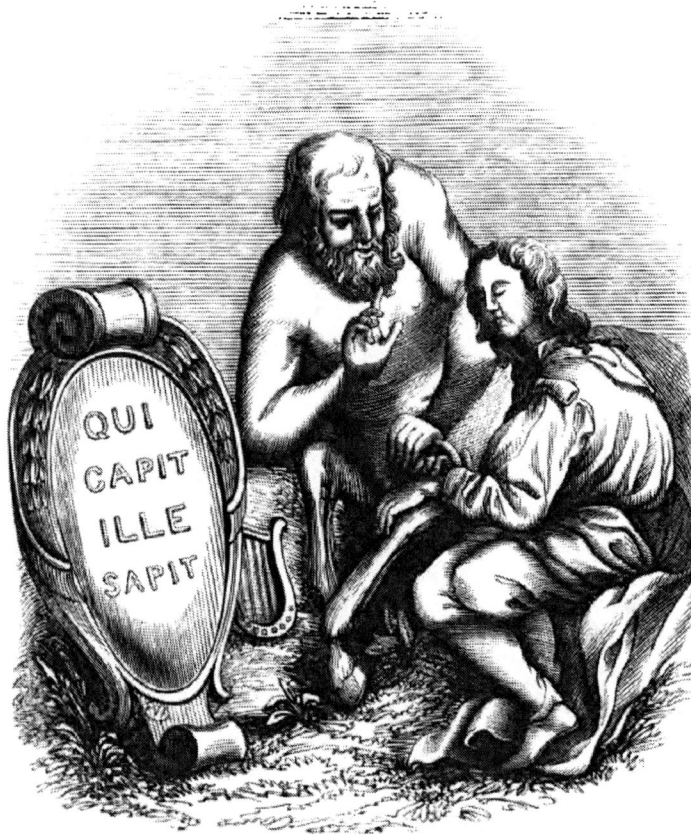

Quæ monstrum? Ille pius CHIRON *Chirurgicus* omnes
Supra Nubigenas, et magni Doctor Achillis.

To make him great, and good, and understand
All things, Old Chiron takes the Youth in hand.
This Horse-man, Hero-trainer, and Bull-baiter
To comprehend, see, *unde derivatur*
The classic Centaur, carrying combined
Animal body and etherial mind;
The link magnetic, though in fable sung,
"Centaur not fabulous," says Dr. Young.

EARLY MAGNETISM.

THE history and philosophies of remote antiquity are laden with a mystery so obscurely fabled, that much of the patience and ingenuity, which the peculiar interest of the subject has from time to time drawn to it, has been wasted, and the keenest intellects have been baffled in endeavouring to penetrate its original idea. The dissatisfaction with which each successive enquirer has regarded the labours of those who have gone before him, and the evident failure of all to interest greatly the general mind, would indicate that the secret intention and universality which, amid all their varied imagery, so sensibly pervades the old mythologies has not been reached, nor the dull spiritless interpretations of modern learning been able to give a voice to the weighty whisperings of their fable lore.

B

We have been content to regard the ancients as strangely fanciful, and to impute to their poets and wisest philosophers such vague and futile imaginings as the least learned amongst ourselves would blush to acknowledge, idly supposing those mystic metaphors and allusions to be without meaning and incomprehensible, which we could not immediately or superficially understand. Thus has it been well said of ancient mythology, that it is like a vintage ill pressed ; we have, indeed, gathered little better than the hulls of the vineyard, having valued but for their clothing the gods of Greece, by their mere names seeking to sanctify our clumsy conceptions, or to such dead original as titles, towns, stars, watch towers and warriors, referring their immortal progeny. the nurtured and educated of old Chiron—that ancient school-master, who, when again venerable as of old he shall go forth instructing, unfolding nature, displaying her occult physics, her mysterious centre, her universal will—in his twofold capacity manifesting, perfecting, shall he not people a new Olympus and herald a golden monarchy once more on earth ?

Then may we cease to congratulate ourselves on the enlightenment of this age, on its practical knowledge and diverse experiments, accumu-

lated with little order and uncertain aim; and
shall not ancient wisdom, so long neglected,
again be eagerly searched out and its sacred
relics appreciated, whilst our levity and profane
interpretation of their holy breath, may teach
humility and draw forth our admiration to its
veriest bounds? For as, by the gradual dawning
upon us of their original light, we are enabled
more and more closely to scrutinize the source
of all obscure tradition, and increasingly to
appreciate the vast intellectual labours and
reputed endowments of our early ancestors, the
less exulting shall we become in the particular
manifestation of the progressive law as respects
ourselves; so indeed, that but for an inborn
hoping faith in ultimate perfection, and the
happy consummation of all things in eternity,
we might rather infer that the chain of universal
existence grows proportionably weaker as it
lengthens out in time.

If wisdom in its completeness has ever existed
or been cultivated in any age or country, Egypt
would be generally acknowledged as the favoured
spot; here, if any where, severe researches were
made into the hidden principles and causes
of things, hence were avowedly derived many
Hebrew mysteries and hence in after times
though secretly and partially, the truth imparted

itself to the master minds of Greece; forming
for them the profound though unavowed source
of that flood of speculation which, with its inner
evidence yet darkly wrapped, has so long been the
veneration of the Western World. Little light
elapsed from the Roman tyranny, and as polite
literature gained gradual ascendency over philosophic pursuit, faith supplied the conviction of
known reality ; and the truth, which again
became concentrated and obscured, was frittered
away in those peripatetical abstractions, the
fallacy of which Bacon so forcibly perceived
and arrested by giving a new impetus to natural
experiment, reducing it to system and scientific
order. But, to use his own expressive words,
truly " this inestimable gift of experience continues to be carried on a slow paced ass;" its
application is yet selfish and desultory; for
science, except in some sensible particulars and
outward adornment, it has done nothing, and
as regards humanity, it is but too evidently
sacrificed to the low and fluctuating nature of
external pursuit ; besides, however well an
abundance of facts may serve to satisfy and
furnish the mere perceptive intelligence, they do
not educate the mind, or evolve that depth and
reality of thought which, with the science of
Universals, has languished and decayed.

But the result of all knowledge, whether of error or of truth, doubtless tends for ever onward, to diffuse the good and send forth its experience into every condition of existence ; so that although our limited sojourn permits us not always to perceive the general design through its cumbrous crust of partial operations, yet as circle after circle passes over and disappears, it leaves behind it, in its ruins, some improved principle on which to renew itself—as thus, though formerly, in its partial and concentrated form, the manifestation of mind was more powerful and brilliant, yet is its diffusion now more generous, stirring, leavening, energizing the general humanity, gaining greater strength as it advances to loosen and remove through every change of opportunity, its long worn fetters of sense and ignorance ; and by these means preparing all, as we would hope, to receive worthily, and with due advantage the free radiation of that living light which has so long been dimly burning and struggling within us ; but which, every surrounding indication now bids us believe, is about to shine forth with an effulgence more than ever heretofore vigorous and unrestrained. Life is everywhere quickening around us ; the world moves onward at a peculiar speed, accelerating as though it neared some

attracting focus ; and, though perchance far yet
within her adytum, the Genius of past wisdom
lies enchanted, the key of her magic treasury is
recovered and known.

It is curious to observe how very gradually
the phenomena, which, from its commencement,
lay hidden in the art of vital magnetism, have
been revealed to individuals, and how tardily
facts which address their reality to every sense
are being received by the public mind. The
world drawn willingly only by the dazzlings of
self-interest, rejects as obnoxious all general and
sudden enlightenment, and avoids, as it would
physical pain, the labour of thought requisite
for the bare reception of a new truth. But
beyond this it is remarkable, that without any
apparent cause, change of intention, or outward
condition, new and admirable manifestations
should have been developed, and always successively, at distant intervals, and never by one
person, or at one time been introduced ; that
Mesmer, though farther advanced than most of
his successors in knowledge of the sympathetic
and curative powers, never induced somnambulism ; and that the phenomena of lucidity
and prevision, now so common, should of themselves, as it were, have followed some time
after the observation of the trance by Puységur.

Be the causes what they may, we have been slowly visited and slowly awakened to the wonders of a new state of life and relationship, to the experience of faculties the very reverse of all we had been accustomed to consider possible, and to an exhibition of power which, while it disturbs the common current of our ideas and eludes reason in its natural search after simple causes, compels the astonished mind to rise as from a long dark dream to look around and think—and who really thinking and looking onward over these passing intervals of doubt and wonderment, has not strange foreshadowings of the coming future, with forebodings full of hope and fear for men and for humanity ? If, without foresight or human intention, revelations so important have already presented themselves, what may we not anticipate as the science advances, surely and rapidly to unfold the hidden allegory of ages before all eyes ?

Let us, if we would shorten our pilgrimage to the shrine of truth, and in our own persons possess right wisdom, glance freely beyond and beneath the slow universal movement and popular sphere of speculation and, (except where benevolence commands our alleviating aid), forsaking the dangerous ground of un-learned experiment, seek from the early erudition

of our inspired forefathers their jealously concealed practice and theoretic knowledge : let us
lay aside the pride of time and prejudice, to look
with combined reverence and scrutiny to the
few records bequeathed us, closely following up
their source through each line and metaphor,
and observing whither they almost exclusively
tend and point. And though there be not yet
granted to us the magic clue of Ariadne, we
have, nevertheless, a sure leading thread by
which we may safely enter, at least, the laby-
rinth of divine philosophy ; and if it fail to
guide us to the inmost temple, yet will it, if
faithfully followed, conduct us to the sacred
approach, and enable us, whilst in some degree
participating, to understand that holy fervour,
aspiration, and awe, with which the high
initiated intellect of all ages has been exalted
and filled ; and to whose regenerate purity and
righteous conception it has sometime been per-
mitted to behold the recondite reality of all
things ; even the beauteous shadow of that High
Archetype, from before whose throne, the rebel
Reason falls for experience; until, having proved
and drunken of the cup of truth, he returns
worshipping, to realise the perfect whole. Let
us then pause, and think, and examine; let us
have a worthy object, and let it be scientifically

and systematically pursued ;—if we would learn the truth of other things, let us seek to know ourselves.

When Bacon bade the searcher of knowledge look outwardly into the maze of the Macrocosm, it was because he saw that the human mind was falsified by sensible images and idols, which refracted the rays of truth ; and at the same time seeing no other natural means of its emerging from this blind condition, but through outward toil and sweat of the brow, he bequeathed to us his " Instrument " to prepare, as he expresses it, a way for the ultimate union, *Mentis et Universi.* For more than two centuries we have possessed this instrument, but have derived from it very indifferent advantage ; whether if its idea had been more legitimately applied, and inductions carried up to first sources, it might have led to the much to be desired goal remains yet to be determined. Meanwhile, having already in our Hands, the far easier link of the artificial trance whereby to *artificial Trance* conjoin the mind to its lost universality, and pass the consciousness regressively through its many phases back to that long forgotten life in reality, may we not venture, with renewed hopes of gain and good fortune, to work once more in the forbidden ground ? And there, whilst applying our energies for internal experience, passing behind the murky media of sense and fantasy, we may find it no presumption to anticipate the day, when we shall behold reflected in the brightened mirror of our own intelligence, the pure truth : not as it may appear individually, or arbitrarily, but in its characteristic necessity and universality.

We would not rashly anticipate nature, or rest satisfied even in the theoretic persuasion, before we have climbed the intermediate spaces and external helps to just inference; but as practical means are often discovered through speculative research, it becomes an important aid towards the fulfilment of truth, and the rational mind works up to and tests its idea. It has been the fashion of modern philosophy to regard humanity from a point of view little dignified, and as holding far lower and less imperial relations to the universe than was in former times alloted to it. Earth-born reason has warred successfully on the Olympic gods; secular fact has taken place of sacred fable, and Divinity has passed out of nature into faith.

The knowledge of antiquity was of a character the very opposite to our own, inasmuch as it was drawn from another spring; whether more or less prolific of truth, may at present rest a matter of opinion; but in endeavouring to explain their writings we have too much overlooked this fact, or, perhaps, have been ignorant of it in its full extent. In order to attain to a knowledge of truth, our earlier ancestors do not appear to have had recourse, like ourselves, to external labour and experiment, but rather to have sought it through its internal experience; they looked on man as a microcosm in which all external things were latent and discoverable. Little regardful of the physiognomy and partial phenomena of nature, they desired to understand her more occult and efficient springs, and this, as is now more than probable, by becoming themselves related to her as a central whole.

Thus do they commonly speak, not as beholding things speculatively, but absolutely in themselves; as comprehending the integral operation of every particular in that great chain of universal cause which, dependent from the Supreme Will, deifies existence, whose every link is an efficient reason, and whose whole is the perfection of all manifested being; and treating on these sublime subjects with infinitely more perspicacity and apparent exactness than would be possible from any exterior source, or to any mere ordinary condition of intelligence.

Thus is it related of the great Proclus that, after passing the preparatory initiations, he was enabled to proceed to the mystic discipline of Plato, and by the help of his preceptor Syrianus, " to survey in conjunction with him, in orderly progression, truly divine mysteries ; that he made a very great progress in a very little time, and from such discipline he increased wonderfully in virtue, as well as in science." His biographer, Marianus, in the following remarkable passage, shows how he gradually proceeded, " throwing aside the instruments of sense as vain, repressing, also, all energies through these instruments, and liberating the soul from the bonds of generation." He then adds, " Proclus made a proficiency in these virtues, as it were, by certain mystic steps, recurring from these to such as are more telestic, being conducted to them by a prosperous nature and scientific discipline. For being now purified, rising above generation, and despising its thyrsus-bearers, he was agitated with a divinely inspired fury about first essences, and became an inspector of the truly blessed spectacles which they contain; no longer collecting discursively the science of them, but surveying, as it were, by simple intuition, and beholding, through intellectual energies, the paradigms in a divine intellect, assuming a virtue which ought to be called wisdom, or something still more venerable than this. The philosopher, therefore, energizing according to this virtue, easily comprehended all the theology of the Greeks and Barbarians, and that which is adumbrated in mythological fictions, and brought it into light to those who are willing and able to comprehend it."

It is further observed by Marianus of this gifted and extraordinary man, that not only did his body possess great symmetry, but a living light, as it were, beaming from his soul, was efflorescent in his person, and shone forth with an admirable splendour which it is impossible to describe; that when lecturing his head was perceived to be surrounded with light, and his eyes to be filled with a fulgid splendour, and the rest of his face to participate of divine illumination: that, furthermore, being purified in an orderly manner by the Chaldean purifications, Proclus became an inspector of the Hecatic visions, as he himself somewhere mentions in his writings. By opportunely moving likewise a certain Hecatic spherula, he procured showers of rain, and freed Athens from unseasonable heat. Besides this, he stopped an earthquake, and other like instances of his power are recorded, as also of Pythagoras, Appollonius, Virgil, Iamblicus, and many of the Platonic successors.*

> " High above æther, there with radiance bright,
> A pure immortal splendour wings its flight :
> Whose beams divine with vivid force aspire,
> And leap resounding from a fount of fire.
> Lo ! on my soul the sacred fire descends,
> Whose vivid power the intellect extends ;
> From whence, far beaming thro' dull body's night,
> It soars to æther decked with starry light,
> And with soft murmurs, thro' the azure round,
> The lucid regions of the gods resound."

Thus moving in ecstatic unison with the celestial spheres, the classic mind sung in the beholding of Universal Being, imaging out its inspirations into free and elegant story. The psychical powers, moving in symphony with the Muses' choir, disposed the whole mind into harmonious measure. The magic world of volition was unfolded; and high in the etherial concave of Intelligence, all Nature was beheld in her deific Exemplar.

> " Felices animæ ! Quibus hæc cognoscere primum
>   Inque domos superas scandere cura fuit,
> Credibile est illos pariter, vitiisque jocisque
>   Altius humanis exeruisse caput."

But gods are not born of sensible conditions,

* See Taylor's Introd. to his Translation of Proclus on the Theology of Plato. *Thomas Taylor*

nor their energies displayed in fettered wills and
imaginations; to the freed essences of mind
alone are they truly present, developing their
orderly processions to assimilated intellect, com-
prehensive of the power and glory of the Whole.
If, then, we would hope to taste anew the exaltation and living beauty of the Antique Muse,
we must break the enchantment which isolates
us in creation; and, emulously passing in order
the silent, initiatory, mystic rites, and rekindling
our lamp at the sacrificial altar, assemble once
again the Supreme Court on Mount Ida in all
its classic strength and magnificence:

"Sume *fidem* et *pharetram,* fies manifestus Apollo.
Accidant capiti *cornua,* Bacchus eris."

"Tunc ire ad mundum archetypum sæpe atq. redire
Cunctarumq; Patrem rerum spectare licebit."

Moved into this shadowly existence, and
drawn away from a knowledge of substantial
cause by the external reference of our whole
being, we are connected with nature's surface,
image, and effects, only by our senses. We
talk of Power and of Spirit indefinitely, and in-
essentially, from negative perceptions of what
they are not, without knowing, or even thinking
of what they are. We are troubled in names
and appearances as the balances of nature
change, and her forms become occult, or mani-

fested to sense ; all is changed and transmuted outwardly in this world, but nothing is destroyed or lost, because of the immutability of its efficient root.   In the centre of all and each existence is its true being and substance from whence it radiates into surface manifestation ; thus the compound crust of matter is not true body, but its vehicle.   Is not WILL the simple substantiality of all things ; the *omnia in omnibus* unparticled, homogeneous, one, in and above all created things ; the causal universal agent, and fountain of all multiform Idea, imparting itself shadowly into creation, and by generation into life ?

Will

The Mind rightly disciplined and related to the Universal, becomes universalized and one with the great magnetic Will of nature ; and revolving with the Infinite Medium through all its spheres, developes in order its various correspondencies, with the regular coadaptation and harmony of its parts ; thence by participation it perceives all things in all, and in itself microcosmically, until at length, becoming perfectly converted to its Principle, the divinized Epitome moves with demiurgic power and grace.

Every living creature has its cause in itself,— the first cause of its own individuality ; but by the particular trespass of self-activity for manifestation, all things are by necessity of conse-

Fall

quence cut off from the monadic rest. A mystery is here unspeakable; this fall, we are to believe, is expiable and through man alone: passed by discipline through the ordeal of Wisdom and essential fire, the passive personality collapses from its circumferential and phenomenal life into that central Omnipresence whose circumference is not.

The Journey

Herein, too, may we have solved for us the problem of free will; not, indeed, that motiveless chimera which human fancy has sometimes loved to frame, but the ancient all-producing Titan freed from death, and the enchantment of his earthly parent to be the Magnet of the mind. As the flame to the coal, so the effect to its cause, in perpetual manifestation, self-motive, and eternal for ever more.

Free will

Thus much is said and thus imperfectly developed, these suggestions are entrusted to fate for their further unravelment, and effects on the good and enlightened mind that may peruse these pages; "*Nucleum esse qui vult, nucem frangat oportet.*" The thoughtless and the vicious are, at present, too deeply busied in worldly interests and machinations to take much heed of speculative truth, even though it were declared to be the fruit of observation; they are yet content to sleep, and pass on from dream to

Sleep & dream

c

dream, forgetting the vanity of the last farce they took a part in, whilst eagerly preparing for the next. And so it is well; this is the befitting time for the Genius of good to lay aside her long indolence, and to bestir herself; she is now called upon for active duty, to counteract, by one well conducted effort, the widely spread energies of vice and ignorance; and rallying round her banner all her many silent votaries, to secure by pre-occupation a science that should be especially her own.

Science confers, or rather reveals, power only; it neither improves, purifies, nor is a blessing of itself; but has its impress of good or evil stamped by its administration and the motives which carry it into act; thus, in proportion to the greatness, is the danger of a gift, and each new light as it opens, lays on us its burden of responsibility.

The whole activity and effort of nature is towards the law of Equilibrium; a preponderance is no sooner established, than variously by her winds, her rains, or lightnings, she hastens to restore the lost balance; her will is drawn constantly, for she loves to fill all things with the plenitude which is in herself. Here below it is her pleasure to fluctuate, to do, and to undo, and never to rest perfectly; but in her

Heaven is the fulfilment of the Law; here justice
is imaged in the balance of symmetrical beauty,
whose equipoise no wanton will dare violate, or
curiosity profane; even for the attempt, mortals
have shared the accursed confusion with the
offending giants in the shades of night.

Everything that is gained by the hand of man,
in the power of his own will, is borrowed and
lost in something else: his weight is not just
because not of the universal; the universal
alone can work justly through man. In the
ordinary conditions of life, this infinite will can
hardly be said to be revealed, and men's actions
are, therefore, necessarily of themselves, and
their wills partake of their own character, whether good or evil; but being comparatively
inoperative and dead, their motion disturbs only
temporarily the balances of nature; but when
launched into the spontaneity of participated
efficience, the self-activity must be in abeyance,
and restrained constantly by the Law which then
moves in it. And here is the discretionary 'Good + Evil
temptation—the forbidden fruit with its choice
of good or evil.

The will of the Magnetiser passing through
the celestial medium to his patient, is, in comparison to our ordinary experience, very effica-
cious; it has, however, this advantage merely

c 2

from moving into a free nature, the intervening firmament of mind ; being itself, in respect of all else, bound as ever in its human shackles. It may be well to observe, by the way, that we should take especial care in experiments of this sort, one on another, remembering that a vacuum is inevitably created somewhere by those who wilfully trifle with the Magnetic trance, and which must, in due time, be expiated in its effects. |Faith,| that spontaneous faith which flows freely from the well-intentioned mind, will be found a far better and more healing influence through the *passes* than any energy of will, benevolent though it be. Let none presume to play idly with so great a blessing as is now restored to us ; for if we do so, and ungratefully degrade its high origin to selfish ends, we may beware lest with the keys of Heaven, we unlock the easier gates of Hell.

One of the greatest evils of national polytheism consists in the licence which it seems to have afforded to the vulgar mind, to particularize its worship for self-proposed ends. Every object that springs from selfish desire, is a false god, a deification of our own will, which being isolated, is ignorant of the universal good, and breaks its operation in as far as it is able. Every prayer that is defined by our own blind will is

[handwritten margin note: Warning about using the magnetic trance incorrectly]

evil and idolatrous, because it does not co-
operate with the general design and will of the
Omniscient Good and equilibrium of existence.
And this is one principle of that perfect self-
submission and humility which is so forcibly
taught us in the precept and example of the
Divine Founder of Christianity. But true unity
of worship with us is yet a name, at most a
creed, and if to worship be in spirit and in truth
to serve, we have more gods in our own passing
follies and base passions, than all the mythologic
list of Greece supplies.

" And in our mental world what chaos drear,
What forms of mournful, loathsome, furious mien,
O ! when shall that eternal morn appear,
These dreadful forms to chase, this chaos dark to clear ?"

" How is the gold become dim ! How is the
most fine gold changed!" the oil of the tabernacle is poured out at the top of every street.
How different were the times, and how different
the mind that formerly wielded the Hermetic
wand ! When the one great object of all discipline was strong enough to bear the body
through the severest tortures, and truth and
virtue were to themselves their own sufficient
goal ; when five long years of unbroken silence,
arduous contemplation, fasting, and prayer, were

scarcely thought sufficient purification for those who aspired to be initiated into the esoteric school. These were no infidels to their convictions, nor dared they wear the cross in practical idolatry, to make religion's pretext cloak a worldly mind and aim. But it may be, that their toil is deemed unwise, their labour fruitless. We think that without their penance we have got their prize; but alas, no! We are, it is true, awarded above our deserts; but so were they—the fervent, wrapped, crucified adorers of the one only Good.

Professing, indeed, ourselves a purer faith, but little understanding its vital ground and conviction; we have misprized these men as pagans and polytheists,—these who, at least, felt the mediatorial necessity, and bearing the divine cross in patience and practical humility, looked forward with confiding hope to its manifested consummation. But every thing bearing relation to the inner life is obscure to the unrelated mind, and by seeking their interpretations outwardly and afar off, we have entirely perverted the idea of ancient theosophy and its sacred fables. " It would not be difficult," says an early writer on this subject, " to show that fables are divine from those by whom they were employed; for they were used by poets, agitated by divinity,

by the best philosophers, and by such as disclose
initiatory rites. In oracles also fables are em- *Initiatory rites*
ployed by the gods ; but why fables are divine
is the part of philosophy to investigate ; fables
assert to all that there are gods, but who they
are, and of what kind, they alone manifest to
such as are capable of so exalted knowledge."
For there is a wide difference between the arbitrary notions of individuated mind, and the
intuitions of divine intellect ; between mythology, degraded by modern commentators, and
the mystical allegory of universal truth. Has
not the most important doctrine in all ages been
delivered in parables and obscure types? And
if these metaphoric rays have dazzled and
bewildered our feeble intelligence, how can we
hope, by our unaided vision, to penetrate to, or
endure their internal light? Unless we can
ourselves become related to its developing condition, how can we expect to unravel the intri-
cacies of early theogony, or without new means
and media to comprehend philosophies and
revelations, professedly emanating from the
fountain of Divinity itself? Are not all first
truths essentially occult ; or, if we think otherwise, is it not because we do not well know or
consider them ? Believing we know many things,
yet understanding nothing, we are doubly igno-

rant; and time bears on wearily the burden of a mystery.

Many elaborate treatises have been put forth with a view to mortalize the spirit of ancient fable; it has been learnedly traced from age to age and from country to country, and its origin laid in remote occurrences and external analogies, political, moral, astronomical, agricultural; or otherwise, as the interpreting genius may have inclined; but, although their universality has admitted and made specious every superficial view, yet their real allusion may not so readily meet the eye; we have searched widely and remotely for interpretations, too little suspecting the constant origination and proximity of their source. Has not the learned Jacob Bryant * sufficiently shown the fabulous being of all early heroes, and the manifest inconsistency of those poetical narratives concerning them; from which, Herodotus, Strabo, and mankind after them, have dated events and fixed as real eras in the world's history? The expedition of the Argonauts, for whom Chiron formed the sphere †

* Analysis of Ancient Mythology. Three vols. 4to.

† The constellation Argo which is so far down in the Southern hemisphere, as to have been certainly invisible to the alleged course of that expedition, for whose especial use it was said to have been originally framed.

which has so puzzled Newton and Dr. Rutherford; the adventures of Theseus, Perseus, Hercules, Dionysius, with a host of others of like import, the Trojan war, and wanderings of Ulysses; are not all these plainly and entirely by him, proved to be inventions founded in no external actuality? Does not all traditionary antiquity bear an impress of allegory, rather than of true history; is it not, perhaps, rather intended to image than to veil reality, to convey idea than to colour facts and mystify occurrences? The symbols, ceremonies, and demigods of all times, have too much analogy one with another, and been too universally admitted in all countries, not to have a deeper root in humanity than it has been in these latter ages the custom to give them credit for; and there are yet concealed, under the imperfect remains of their imagery, great, fundamental, vital, and forgotten truths.

Some persons have been alarmed by finding that the rites and mysteries of the Hebrews were similar to those of prior and cotemporary nations; thinking it might seem to insinuate a borrowed source, and thereby deprive them of their sacred authority; but this judgment appears quite groundless; their truth on the contrary, is rather strengthened than otherwise, by the fact of their universality. Religious creeds and modes of worship may indeed change, or be borrowed by one people from another; but their base in reality is immutable, and always originates where it is rightly understood. We have little faith in mere individual revealments, it is irrational to. suppose that any mind was ever truly inspired with exclusive principles; truth does not belong to persons or periods, but according to the purity of the conditions, and universality of the conception is the extent and nature of its inspiration. How much infidelity has sprung from the long obscuration of sacred truths; how then can it hardly be mischievous that we have once more given to us a means for unfolding them? A clearer understanding and experience of them will ultimately range all good and reasonable minds on their side; and their general confirmation will rejoice the confiding believer.

The Egyptian authority has been everywhere highly venerated, but their hieroglyphics are evidently too esoteric for profane scrutiny to unriddle; their philosophers generally chose the symbolical in preference to the fabulous mode of clothing their doctrine; and as it is probably the deepest, so do we find it the most dark of all, and the study has always proved bewildering and unsatisfactory in the extreme. We have few relics left of Egyptian learning, and these, probably, none of the most important, for her priests were for a long period the oracles of the world; and if from her smothered embers, the Greeks were able to kindle so bright a flame: what must have been her glory when she flourished as a nation, and wisdom was at the zenith of her excellence and magic power.

> " O quam te dicam bonam
> Antehac fuisse; tales cum sint reliquiæ!"

O mother of the ART! O land of CHAM! Egypt

That the Egyptian remains have special magnetical allusion, has been observed by many authors on this subject; but little has yet been gleaned concerning their practice, except that it must have differed in many respects from our own. It is frequently observable that the three first fingers only of the hand are extended, the Fingers other two being bent down on the palm, and in some figures even designedly broken off; this is the case in the Indian idols, who, with their many arms and hands are always in magnetical postures. Each finger has its different

Fingers cont

hieroglyphic; the whole hand is generally extended for healing or blessing; but when the image is rather of will or power, the thumb and two first fingers only are employed.* The general impression conveyed by their symbols is mystical and sacred, and more seldom curative. The animals they worshipped were probably in no ordinary state of being, but had become, as they considered, divinized by being moved into and under the universal will.

* We would here note too, the mysteries of the Dactyli Idæi (literally the fingers of Mount Ida) so celebrated amongst the Greeks and Asiatics, and concerning which mythological personages, Strabo and Diodorus, give particular account. The Cretans paid them divine honours for having nursed and brought up Jupiter, whence some suppose them to have been the same as the Corybantes and Curetes; accounts, however, vary, and concerning their number some say they were ten; five brothers, and as many sisters; others, that like the horned Centaurs there were one hundred of them who worked together at the foot of Mount Ida. They are said to have been magicians, and addicted to mystical ceremonies, and that Orpheus was their disciple and carried their mysteries into Greece; that, moreover, "the Dactyli of Asia were peculiarly famous for their skill in the healing art, so that their name indeed was synonymous with that of the Healers." Diodorus relates that they surprised the people of Samothracia with an exhibition of their wonders during the initiatory rites, which consisted in trials more or less strong adapted to the capacity of the aspirants.

The Arkite mysteries, so anciently celebrated in this and most other Gentile nations, were obviously, from the accounts transmitted to us, strangely and practically significative of the saving and renovating power of the universal Spirit, variously personified as Isis, Ceres, Damater, Minerva, Archia, Beroe, &c. The stay in the ark was bewailed as a state of temporary death, and the going forth, which was accompanied with mystic foretokens, was hailed as a re-birth and purification not dissimilar in idea from our baptismal form. All the heroes are reported to have passed through an experience of this kind, and to have gained some great object by the passage; they were many of them said to be originally born at Thebes, which was a name of the ark, as also Arkeus, or Archeus. A little attention to derivations may serve to clear many minor difficulties; for there are diverse manifestations, though but one spirit reigning paramount through and over all, the fountain of divine life and light, *Magna Deum Mater*, and restoring ordeal of all created things.

> " Æon came near, the sage of ancient days,
> Æon, a prophet famed, who gently reached
> His aged hand to Beroë, and withdrew
> The veil of justice which obscured her brow,

Then loosened all her bands; Æon had seen
Age after age in long succession roll,
But, like a serpent which has cast his skin,
Rose to new life in youthful vigour strong.
Such the reward which Themis gave the man
Washed in her healing waters."

The philosophic mythology of Greece is
wholly free from the objections which poetic
licence has cast upon the generally accepted
story of its gods; the freedom and irony of
which has given a handle to prejudice, and,
unfortunately, thrown a slur over the whole.
But, extravagant as are many of its conceptions,
and far out of the common road of thought,
yet have we no good reason to consider them as
altogether fanciful, or even in their kind inexact.
Truth casts its allegory, as do objects their
shadow, in the sun-light, gracefully deformed.
It would be easy to expatiate on this subject,
and bring forward particular evidence as to the
references of many of the old writers; but in
the present state of science and incredulity of
the public mind, it might be premature and
inexpedient, independently of the hazard of
wearying the reader with unfamiliar reflections,
and details which would now, perhaps, be considered as irrelevant or uninviting.

But not poetry itself has ever reached, much

less exaggerated the surpassing reality; and for those to whom such inquiries may still be attractive, or who have had the glowing and more true impressions of early youth unwillingly disappointed by the cold externality of our learned commentators, a deeper and more purely allegorical consideration of classical tradition, may be grateful and encouraging to further research; for the subject becomes more and more alluring as it opens, exalting and extending the ranges of thought, our hopes are renewed of beholding for ourselves its well-spring of truth; and in it reflected, the promise of a new existence for man, with the image of a happier and yet unseen world;

> " Though from our birth the faculty divine
> Is chained and tortured, cabbin'd cribb'd, confin'd,
> And bred in darkness, lest the truth should shine
> Too brightly on the unprepared mind,
> The beams pour in; and time and skill will couch the
> blind."

The occult spring of mystic allegory moves as we apply the master-key; the first door opens, and we stand once more on the threshold of nature's laboratory. Secret knowledge is now becoming public; sacred mysteries may be revealed to the profane, and truths long since

wrapped in hieroglyphics and buried in pyra-
mids, be declared in the common type and in the
common tongue. There have been those who
have dreaded this day, and anticipating its
coming, have prophecied sadly and seriously
respecting it ; nor is the spirit now dead that
formerly dictated secresy in these matters. The
entire causes of such cautions may as yet be
unknown, or but dimly perceived, even by those
practically acquainted with the nature of magnetism ; but they who carelessly rank its revealments and consequences amongst the many discoveries and mere inventions of the day, have
thought little and superficially, as time will
show.

It is, however, no less irrational than painful
to dread the results of inevitable enlightenment,
for we cannot see far or clearly enough into
consequences to justify mistrust in the provident
necessity of nature and events as they take
place ; and now that the flood-gates are irre-
versibly opened, we must, with all faith in
humanity, encourage the stream to flow freely
onward, so that all may become instructed as
fully and as quickly as possible ; and increased
knowledge be thus made to direct a power which
no external coercion can secure or suppress,
and that the restraint, (if such it must be called

which prevents the doing of evil), may be found in the exaltation of our moral nature; for outward laws, as respects this, must continue as they ever have been unavailing, since they cannot arrest or determine the secret will. The protective power and beneficial impulse are implanted within us; where they are dormant they must be aroused, and obvious interest every where prevent abuse, for man holds a power that forbids him to be the enemy of his fellow, and the facts now unfolding must moralize the world.

Vast truths have been declared to us, and many facts transmitted which, we being ignorant of their ground of possibility, have disbelieved and neglected; though in many instances we may now observe, the great amount of intelligent testimony should have taught more diffidence, as supporting mere vain fables, it would be as a greater wonder, than that the said fables should prove to be unexplained truths. But it is not to modern pride and ignorance alone that the loss of so much valuable knowledge is to be imputed; for the special policy of the Ancients respecting it has doubtless contributed not a little to this remarkable retrogression. The priests of all religions holding such science as their especial prerogative,

D

and being well aware that with it they held exclusive power, were mutually interested in with-
holding it from the people ; and this motive, together with their vigilant training, secret initia-
tion, and life-bound oath, conspired with the
bond of power to enforce fidelity and render
them watchful and ingenious in finding means
to prevent its diffusion out of their own body.
Learned men, if not exactly guided by priestly
motives, have been nevertheless influenced by
them ; the dread of envy and persecution, with
certain conscientious fears of the results that
might arise from showing to the ignorant truths
which they were ill prepared to receive, and to
the immoral, powers which they might fearfully
abuse, induced them to employ abstruse terms
in dead languages, with passages of hidden or
double meaning ; and for the entire veiling of
the deeper esoteric experience, and securing of
exoteric mystery, they had recourse to particular
hieroglyphics and cabalistic signs. These sacred
sciences have nevertheless existed in all ages,
and been successively revived or degraded according to the hands into which they have
fallen ; principles having at intervals been
neglected, and low means only retained and
resorted to by inferior minds, they have fallen
into contempt, becoming proscribed as vile and

magical; whilst their professors, mere " artizans of miracles," have debased their profession, until at length, scepticism set its seal on all wonders, and miracles were suppressed by opposed convictions.

We may find on investigation that there has been less direct falsehood and more craft in the world formerly than has been generally supposed; and truth artfully veiled has, to simple minds, borne a semblance of falsehood, and been despised as such; thus too we have been led on to extremes of doubt and credulity, according as individual temperament and the fashion of the age may have inclined. But let us not too hastily condemn, as faithless or illiberal, the wary philosophic spirit which, seeing the preponderance of natural evil in the world, and the prevalence of human debasement, has in all ages wrapped in parabolic types the deepest theosophic knowledge; not from any mistrust in it or its legitimate conclusions, but from a dread of its desecration in human selfishness.

. It is true, modern science has been more lavish of her discoveries, but then they lose in import what she gains in liberality; for though she have faithfully served us in her outward sphere, and still on a little while longer may flourish, and boast of her astronomy which has

eclipsed the judiciary astrology of Ptolemy and
Pythagoras, of her experimentalism which has
rendered it impossible to jugglers and sorcerers
any longer to perform miracles, or of her chemistry, which has destroyed the alchemical
chimera; yet what does all this signify? Every
thing intrinsical is hidden from our *mode* of
search; we are experienced only in outward
qualities and accidents; sciences have super-
seded each other in time and locality, and we
have been prone to contemn those which we
could neither attain to or understand. Taken
in the aggregate, the modern study of mankind
has not been mán; and herein do our opinions
and conclusions most widely differ from those
of the Ancients with whom the NOSCE TE IPSUM
regulated the thoughts and efforts of the greatest
minds, all other indeed being esteemed secondary and worthless in comparison.

The meagreness and insufficiency of our philosophy becomes daily more apparent, and facts
press us fast onward to seek anew from nature
an explanation of her marvels; it is not the
superstitious alone who pervert facts to favour
their prejudices: as often is sophistry found
under the mask of philosophy, and nature herself warped and misrepresented to suit the individual judgments and assertions of those who

discard, indeed, supernatural interposition, but to supply it with arbitrary or insufficient causation ; and who though weak in faith, are sceptically credulous, and so often choose the harder side. Reason must exert herself afresh ; for if she pass not quickly the barrier within which partial observation has held her, she will cease to triumph as heretofore, in many minds, over vulgar experience ; we have warred long enough with internal instincts, traditions, and even with the impressions of sense when these have not fallen in with our ideas of rationality ; and in very faithlessness have degraded science, and given her over to the service of those petty projects and small interests which have practical sway in this sensible world.

Though the more refined operations of nature are hidden from our obtuser senses, they need not be from our understanding ; we are not incapable of at least an intellectual appreciation of those finer agencies which escape common susceptibility, and are sensibly manifested only in the effects. Influences, however apparently subtle, are only so relatively to less refined subjects ; for things are affected by their similars ; that which is gross affects outward sense, that which is mental, cerebral sense ; and so on even to the finest projections of reason towards

Intelligibles ; by which we are mentally carried
back to the *superstantial* in all things. The less
grossly palpable any body is, the more simple
and essentially potent does it become. "*Maxima
de nihili visitu fulgura fiunt.*" All observation, in
short, tends to refine our notions, not only of
causal being, but of its unfolding into physical
action ; passing the disputed question of the
materiality of mind or powers of thinking, we
are led to speculation on the essentiality of thought
itself; from conjectures concerning the natural
generation and mechanical suggestion of ideas
in the brain, to their fixed entity, actual ema-
nation, and constant transmission to distant
objects.

> "Illis viva acies, nec pupula parva, sed ignis,
> Trajector nebulæ, et vasti penetrator operti."

All perceptions perhaps require to be experienced in some degree before their idea can
be truly conveyed, or their verbal expression
become quite intelligible ; but once forced by
observation beyond the limits of ordinary experience, it matters little how far ; as whatever
phenomena present themselves, inscrutable
though they be by present knowledge, we are
assured they do not transgress the order of
nature. Have we not facts of transportive

imagination enough to satisfy the boldest poetic fancy, or the ardent eloquence that long since declared that man contains within him all the powers of nature; from his being, as a centre, bearing relation to the whole, the universe is reflected in his little world.

The multitude, unpractised in matters of subtle reasoning and speculation, are incapable of perceiving aright any thing except as it outwardly affects them; in practical appliances they always go astray, in default of the first movement of the leading few; the pioneers are the responsible conductors of the march; and the early enlightened advocates of Mesmerism may, all more or less if they be active and earnest, image out into its general application the good which each individually desires.

The power of the operator's will in changing the dispositions and habits of the sleepwaker, (though for reasons above offered, very dangerous ground for experiment), cannot, *as a fact*, be too well noted; it is a true, though feeble and partial type of the renovating power of that all-pervading, educating, disciplining, purifying, Vital Spirit, which in former ages of the world was dignified with the name of Wisdom; and of whose concentrated power all our external efforts for progress and amendment are but the dead and comparatively ineffective shadows.

" Sed fortasse aliquis quærit, sapientia quid sit,
Nil aliud certe est, nisi prima scientia per quam
Mens pura, et nullo mortali pondere pressa,
Libera terrenis affectibus, atria cœli
Scandit, et etheriâ cum diis versatur in aulâ,
Omnia despiciens prorsus mortalia tanquam
Frivola, et assiduè tendens velut ignis in altum."

Book " Such," says M. Gauthier, speaking on this point, " such are the unheard of benefits of magnetism, that faults which were excessively prominent previous to the somnambulic state, no longer existed in the awakened patient."*

For such observations as these the science of phrenology may be available; as, if the intention gradually works itself into manifestation through the organism, as might be expected, corresponding changes of development may be fairly and satisfactorily tested. Considered as a collection of inductive facts, few will probably now presume to deny the eminent usefulness and truth of phrenology; but the zeal of some of its advocates has certainly been over and above, in claiming for it exclusive authority in

* See *Traité Pratique du Somnambulisme*. A. Gauthier. Paris, 1843.

mental science. Without by any means sup-
plying, or being able to supply, the place of the
elder metaphysics, phrenologists have openly
condemned and set aside its labours, and that
in a sphere of observation eminently above their
own. By its very external nature, phrenology
can never become definite enough to appreciate
the finer manifestations, much less the essential
laws of mind which consciousness reveals to us ;
and admitting that consciousness is liable to
err in individuals—is not sensible observation so
too ? But when metaphysicians err, it is not
so much in consciousness, for this in its depth
is uniform in all, but in their inferences and
conclusions drawn by the partial and contingent
nature of reflective reason ; and to this objection
phrenology is also open in common with all
objective science. The assertion of some phrenologists that their " discovery has supplied the
great desideratum of metaphysical accuracy and
precision," is a very singular and grave mistake.
Accuracy and precision do not belong to such
manifested particulars and unstable system of
organs, as phrenologists dispute about even
amongst themselves. All experimental fact,
and this from its relations above all, is to be
respected ; but when carried above its ground,
it is in danger of becoming empirical, vaunting

itself to the prejudice of investigations above the limits of its capacity.

The internal principles about which metaphysics are conversant, the relations and associations of ideas, in short all experience in subjectivity can only, if at all, be reached by the mind in abstract contemplation of itself; that which we need is the right image and revelation, and this we shall obtain when the true conditions are supplied. Now it is believed, and on no light evidence, that the magnetic trance affords, nay, is itself, when justly and perseveringly ordered for that end, THE METAPHYSICAL CONDITION, pre-eminently perfect. It removes the sensible obscuration, and presents a clearer glass before the mind than it can ever regard in the natural state. The patient is no sooner lightly entranced, than he begins to feel an internality never before known to him, and which may be increased with more or less effect according as the intention is fixed, and the calibre of the minds and circumstantial conditions are favourable or otherwise; though under the simple ordinary operation of one agent and patient, the work will hardly become universal. "Take first the beam from out thine own eye, and then thou shalt see clearly to remove the mote which is in thy brother's eye."

" Non bene tractantur musæ prope perque fenestras
    Vix in sole solent, atque valere foro ;
Nec mediâ ridere dic, vel luce favere,
    Sol lux ac homines ad joca multa trahunt
Sic præunda forum, sudum simul atque plateæ
    Major et e musis tunc quoque messis erit."

That the Pythagoreans, Platonists, and all the intellect of that time, had recourse to this mode of vision is now very evident from their writings ; and however much their systems may appear to vary in particulars, they had <u>one esoteric root</u>, in which they all by co-knowledge agreed, and by means of which they gained higher elevation in science, with more melody of thought and eloquence for its expression than we, with all our labours and enlightenment, have ever dreamed of, or had capacity to appreciate. For these could compel <u>the Muses' inspiration</u>, and move the spheres to give it birth ; for them the Olympic gods assumed their deity, and all the heroes their mighty labours. In their Hand was the power of all experience, the including firmament of every space, the nucleus of all things to be unfolded in time. <u>Chiron</u> prepared them for the Elysian Heaven, or <u>Charon</u> wafted them to the Tartarean shades ;

" PALMAque nobilis,
   Terrarum dominos
   Evehit ad deos !"

" Hæc via scintillans sublustri nocte retecta,
Innumeris nitido cælo rutillissima stellis,
Sapphirina cluet sat cognita frondibus ipsis,
Manibus hoc iter est felices ad arva palati
Secretumque thronum noctuque diuque piorum,
Succensis genium facibus celebrantur hypœthræ ;
Hæc siquidem locus est, quem sides jura poesi,
Haud timeam sedes divûm dixisse senatûs."

To a mind merely practical, every universal
proposition appears abstract, because it does not
regard the true nature of things ; yet were it
not for these so styled abstractions, we should
be inevitably plunged in the abyss of Pyrrho-
nism. Every conclusion of reason has its evidence in faith : that is to say, all inquiry rests
in a universal idea, a fundamental axiom of
mind, without appeal ; we believe in these as we
believe in our own identity, simply because we
cannot do otherwise ; the laws of demonstration,
mathematical for instance, are primary and
spontaneous, subsisting by virtue of their own
inherent necessity. These ideas, though they
may seem to be first excited by, cannot be derived from sense ; they are laws of causality,
perfect in themselves, prior to, and determining
all sensible particulars ; and we dare not question the last grounds of their intuition ; they are
the natural revelation of the λoγoς in man, the
light which lightens every man that cometh

into the world. Reflective reason is personal, reason + intuition
partial, and erring ;—divine intuition is impersonal, universal, and can never err.

"In truth," observes Fénélon, "my reason is Fenélon
in myself, for it is necessary that I should continually turn inward upon myself in order to
find it; but the higher reason which corrects
me when I need it, and which I consult, is not
my own, it does not make specially a part of
myself. Thus, that which may seem most our
own, and to be the foundation of our being, I
mean our reason, is that which we are to believe most borrowed. We receive at every
moment a reason superior to our own, just as
we breathe an air which is not ourselves. There
is an internal school, where man receives what
he can neither acquire outwardly for himself
nor learn of other men who live by alms like himself." Thus is the supreme reason found to rule in
all things universally; as in man made manifest,
beyond the control or modifying energy of his
personal will, fixed, fontal, and everlasting.

It is a truth admitted by metaphysicians,
that if the Absolute be without the sphere of
possible knowledge, philosophy must be always
regarded as a mere phenomenal and delusive
pursuit. To this last conclusion, however, the

human mind is naturally very loth to assent, and many and ingenious are the theories by means of which it has endeavoured to assure to itself a capacity above ordinary conditions and modes of thought; yet every supporter of the positive side of the question has had his successful objectors on the other, so that the matter yet rests, and is much despaired of by the general reason of mankind.

That a truth so necessary as to be instinctively present in every mind, and as inferentially involved in the fact of outward existence, as the unit is concluded from its dependent plurality, should be denied as an affirmative to human reason may at first consideration appear strange and improbable ; yet so it is : by the *transitive activity* of individual thought, it is precluded from a *positive* knowledge of the essential unity towards which it tends.

The knowledge which is absolutely one, cannot be attained in the personal consciousness, since this, by the necessity of its participated nature, is only cognizant under an antithesis of subject and object ; and thus conditionated, beholds itself and all other things only as relative phenomena, that is, as they appear imaged by itself to itself, and never in simple identity of thought and being. The Absolute, being but one, and its knowledge consequently but one, can be truly known only *in* itself, the fountain of thought ineffable, subverting all expression. Its shadow, in us, recedes constantly behind the *secondary* unity of our intelligence ; by endeavouring to convey we instantly dismiss it, and by reflecting while yet on the verge of its conception, we annihilate the inspiration.

The German metaphysicians, Schelling more *Schelling* especially, pressed by the difficulties which thus disable the personal consciousness and prevent it from transcending the limits of rational inference, despised its trammels, and relinquishing it and them together, asserted the existence of a higher faculty in man, by which he is enabled to surpass all conscious thought, and come at once into identified relationship with essential being ; a state in which all difference of subject and object becoming merged, the Unconditioned is known absolutely in itself. This sublime capacity of mind, moving one with the Infinite, they have named the Intellectual Intuition.

In order to its refutation, it is said that this species of unconscious intuition is impossible ; because by the annihilation of consciousness, we destroy thought itself, which takes away with it all possibility and imagination of true being : that the Intuition is therefore a chimera, a pure abstraction, and not a real subsistence.

An eminent French author and philosopher, M. Cousin, already awakened to these objections, yet still desirous for the honour of philosophy and innate assent of the human mind, to retain, if possible, the positive ground, has ventured to draw down the Intuition once more into human consciousness, even in its ordinary conditions ; but this effort would seem to have been unsuccessful.* By drawing the pre-existent reality into its posterior image, the theory obscures its own object, and brings about the reverse dilemma of the Intuition, in that it conditionates the unconditioned. How can it be possible for the effect to know its cause in its *separated* individuality, unless it be by inference? Spontaneity of perception, however nearly it may verge, and truly reflect the subjective image, is not in thought co-essentially cognizant ; and simply for this reason, that it is not the ontological unity itself. Thus is it in every way obvious that *the true knowledge* does not supervene " under the apparent relativeness and subjectivity of the principles of thought." For be-

* See an admirable article in the Edinburgh Review. No. 99. Art. 11. ("Cours de Philosophie," par M. V. Cousin.)

hind every particular modification and possibility of individuated consciousness, is yet implied the infinite nucleus of Being and Absolute Will.

If the Absolute is, as itself, to be known independently, and before its manifestation, it is plain to every thinking mind, that it must be by the experience of co-essence in union, not by reason or any reflective act: in short, as has been before said, by the becoming It. " *Nec sentire Deum nisi qui pars ipse Dei est.*"

Thus then, if this species of cognition cannot take place in our *personal* consciousness, and if beyond the pale of consciousness, *being* is annihilate, we must, if we would yet hold fast the anchor, seek some other point of rest, and try if there be not between these extremes some mode of consciousness free from the *duplicity* which incapacitates our own.

We believe by inference, and on the principle of contradiction, that the one *is;* and naturally include, in such idea of essential being, that of consciousness ; which, as pertaining to, or rather being itself the pure subjectivity, can only be thought of consistently with itself, as impersonal, unconditioned, and universal.

Reflective reason rests in the pure abstraction of all relative existence, unable to pass the infinite abyss which opens upon the extreme verge

E

of thought betwixt it and the one: hence though
it is very requisite, as a preliminary aid to relationship, and the right perception of intelligibles, yet it is not, as has been alleged, the
bridge by which we can immediately pass from
Psycology to Ontology, but rather contrariwise;
its self-activity is the last intervening barrier
between them. The positive First and the negative Last, each implying the other unmanifest-
edly throughout the immeasurable procession
of sensible and temporal existence.

☆ The human mind by the various disciplines
and trials of Wisdom, (the term is not here employed vaguely; or intended to be ambiguous)
may become truly based; and from that base,
in pure passivity, be drawn by faith and the
harmonious rest of union into one with All; to
have its vision, through true light, in God, and
know itself in its Creator.

" Ego non sum jam qui fueram, amplius Ego."
(I—no longer myself—AM more.)

The Work   This is the work, this its object, and its end;
the line returns to form the circle into its
beginning; and they join not in time, for their
union is eternity.

In his single human strength, man is unable
to know this; without habitual contemplation,
we cannot even rise above a perceptive possi-

bility of this theoretic and very actual truth:
if, therefore, the idea, here briefly suggested,
of the universalised consciousness being attain-
able by man in ecstatic relationship and collapsed
personality, serve in some degree to clear the
imagination and present to any mind, a less
objectionable image than that which the *Unconscious* Intuition, or *Conditioned* Intelligence
may have afforded, it is all that is aspired to or
at present desired.* Increased belief may be
obtained through contemplation, in that free
perspicacity of thought, which reflects the original in every intelligence. Conviction belongs
alone to that acme of vital conversion which is,
and by its own will and necessity, ever must be,
incommunicable and arcane.

" For the knowledge of it is a most *Divine
Silence*, and a rest of all the senses ; for neither
can he that understands *That*, understand any
thing else, nor he that sees *That*, see any thing
else, nor hear any other thing, nor, in sum,
move the body.

* If, from the natural *personality* of its acceptation, the term
consciousness be yet found inapplicable to the Infinite Idea;
it may be taken merely as intended to convey the closest
image of it, which our ordinary mental condition affords : the
imagination must be cleared, by abstraction, from all *duplicity* in its conceptive shadow of universal being.

E 2

" For, shining steadfastly up, and round about the whole mind, it enlighteneth all the soul, and loosing it from the bodily senses and motions, it draweth it from the body and changeth it wholly into the essence of God."

O marvellous, miraculous consummation! and thou, that by the strange necessity of fate, and undue balance of thy self-born nature, art fallen from the first image in which thou wast created! O man! who, with thyself, hast lost all other things, save one—Behold again the beatific vision, remember, know the Beauty—the true Good—the Heaven of which, thou wast thyself the living type and manifested temple! and after this manner contemplate God; " as having the whole world to Himself, as it were, all thoughts and intellections. If, therefore, thou wilt not equal thyself to God, thou canst not understand God, for the like is intelligible by the like.*

---

* It has occurred since writing the above extract, that this passage might possibly suggest a presumptuous or otherwise erroneous idea to minds unfamiliarised to this sacred subject, and be consequently destructive of the whole tenor and object of these remarks; for nothing is so calculated, or more eminently tends to humble man, as he is, than even a small insight into what he might and ought to be; but it is impossible really to profane the Divine Idea, for it cannot be reached by a profane or unprepared mind; and as the fear of God is the begin-

Belief

Contemplate / Meditate

" Increase thyself into an immense greatness, leaping beyond every body, and transcending Time, become Eternity, and thou shalt understand God. If thou *art able* to believe in *thyself*, that nothing is impossible, but accountest thyself immortal, and that thou canst understand all things, every art, every science, and the manner and custom of every living thing.

If you are able to believe in yourself

" Become higher than all Height, lower than all Depth, comprehend *in thyself*, the qualities of all the creatures, of the fire, the water, the dry, and the moist, and conceive likewise that thou canst at once be every where, in the sea and in the earth. Thou shalt at once understand thyself not yet begotten, in the womb, young, old, to be dead and the things after death, and all these together; as also all times, places, deeds, quantities, qualities, or else thou canst not yet understand God. But if thou shut up thy soul in the body, and abuse it, and say, I understand nothing, I can do nothing, I am afraid of the sea, I cannot climb up into heaven, I know not

shut up the soul in the body

ning of wisdom, so is presumption the end of ignorance: not then by prematurely and irreverently drawing down the Idea, but by piously aspiring, and raising the Conception through graduated links and intellectual media can we ever hope to draw the spectacle of our adoration: by pride man fell, in humility, he will rise, to make manifest all Truth.

who I am, I cannot tell what I shall be; what hast thou to do with God?" for thou canst understand none of these fair and good things; be then a lover of the body and evil.

" For it is the greatest evil not to know God: but to be able to know, and to will, and to hope, is the straight way, and the divine way proper to the Good: and it will every where meet thee, every where be seen of thee, plain and easy, when thou dost not expect or look for it. For there is nothing which is not the image of God. And yet thou sayest, God is invisible, but be advised—for who is more manifest than He? For, therefore, hath he made all things, that by all things, thou mayest see Him.

" This is the good of God, this is his virtue, to appear; there is nothing invisible, no not of such things as are incorporeal;

" For the sleep of the senses is the sober watchfulness of the Mind, and the shutting of the eyes, the true Sight. Let these things, thus far forth, be made manifest unto thee;

" Understand in like manner all other things by Thyself, and thou shalt not be deceived."

" We awaken, from the Intellectual Intuition," says Schelling, " as from a state of death;" and we awaken by reflection into that created perso-nality, wherein, it is impossible any longer to

know Him. The vision, graven in hallowed
memory, is all that remains to us ; for the object
of human reason is the limit of its power ; and
the pure zero of all relative conception waits before
the throne of God.

Nothing is truly imaged in this world any
more than we are ourselves, who do but look
and dream on its falsified circumference ; or like
the people in Plato's book of laws, who lived
satisfied in a city underground, furnished only
through certain apertures with small portions of
dim light. But when some of these fortunately
emerged from their subterranean darkness, and
beheld the beauties of the broad and glorious
day, although they were at first uncomfortably
dazzled by its superior light, they disdained the
fancied felicities of their former dark abode, and
lamented the miseries of their yet imprisoned
friends. And we too, so long immured, are we
not about to emerge into the sunlight ? The
Spirit is full wearied of the long Sabbath which
she has kept in silence, through so many circles
of ages, with the assurance of a great purpose
through her to be wrought out ; the inner mind
struggles for a new birth, to redeem philosophy,

and to make manifest its end, and only object in the purification and perfection of human life.

Milton's Paradise Lost

" Celestial light shine inward and the mind
Thro' all her powers irradiate ; there plant eyes,
All mist from thence purge and disperse, that we
May see and tell of things invisible to mortal sight."*

Our true purpose

★In its first true sense human progression is internal, individual, essential, a moulding of the lower irrational portion of the mind into accordance and obedience to the higher intellectual archetype ; a restoring or building up as it were, of a moral monarchy within, by conviction, constant endeavour, and the moving, organising power of a faithful concentrated and uplifted will.

Our false labors

The advance from a simple savage existence to a complex civilised mode of life, is, in the bare comparison of very equivocal reality. All the many changes, known and recorded, which have taken place about superficials, pass on, leaving us even as they find us in perplexity, missing and mistaking continually the true aim of our own and of all existence ; still labouring and undermining our efforts, as we supply the

* Milton's Paradise Lost.

causal living fountain of human suffering and
delusion which, every where imparting its free
flowing fecundity, plays on securely and unin-
terruptedly within.

> " O sons of earth! attempt ye still to rise
> By mountains piled on mountains to the skies?
> Heaven still with laughter your vain toil surveys
> And buries madmen in the heaps they raise."

To expect or even wish for felicity whilst we
continue to falsify our susceptibilities and sub-
mit to the degrading tyranny of our passions is
mere imbecility; it is looking for effects inversely
to their causes, and hoping not only against all
theoretic possibility, but contrary to our every
intuition of moral utility, justice, and experience.
The obstacles which externals every where present to our selfishness might long since have
taught us how vain is its pursuit: but it would
seem, that as it becomes more obvious, our
folly increases, as if to hide itself in the gloom
that deepens at every step of departure from the
simplicity of truth. And it is this, which has
most to be guarded against in the application of
Magnetism, where, so specifically, the intention
carries and immediately images its principle in
act. Springing directly from ourselves, this
highly effective agent flows forth, as the mind

directs, to good or evil; and imposes, in sure consequences on him who wields it, its inherent accountability.

Few perhaps, observe themselves with sufficient scrutiny to know, how surely they bear the just consequences of their own motives and misdeeds, and how inevitably the canker which false intention lays at the root of an action, however far away its outward consequences may be removed, is essentially felt and expiated at its first source. It is not purposed, in this place, to trouble the reader at large on this subject, neither is it necessary, as the law of conscience and individual experience are far more effective criteria to the generality of minds, than ethical propositions, however, clearly demonstrable; we instinctively know that, however, much good and evil may appear to be incidentally implicated in this world, they each must work their opposite results through every seeming deviation; and that though we may endeavour to serve ourselves and cheat existence in outward relations, we cannot evade the moral law in our own being. Oh! that we could but as consciously feel and obey, as we are able in theory to perceive, the precision of the laws which govern in the moral world, and practically appreciate the mathematical exactness with which natural justice is dealt out to us in time! But we are as spell bound to delusion, and constrained mistrust in ourselves, in one another, in all things, even in the power of Good to work its own right results. No estimate can be made of the sad effects which this cheerless infidel spirit operates throughout society; it dislocates and dishonours every relation in life to which it can reach; our hopes and destinies are forfeited in its abyss, as by a horrible perversity, it degrades reason, binding her to the service of blind sordid impulses, instead of her own clear light.

At the present time when all are more or less eagerly engaged in the pursuance of external advantages and under penalty of being cast into the fiery furnace of the world's scorn, do fall down and worship that earth-born goddess of temporal utility which opinion has set up, it would be vain enthusiasm to attempt to divert attention, but for a moment, from so favoured an idol were it not that in the minds of all, even its most degraded votaries, there already exists a most real and bitter sense of its insufficiency, and latent deformity;—and until Wisdom shall have effected that internal renovation which, above all things we now need, it is vainly that we seek in externals a harmony and happiness which has not been imaged there.—Yet still we

linger on in expectation, and with that abiding
patience, which is the test of faith in a good
cause, may we continue to seek on, not vaguely
as heretofore, for passing excitements, but with
steadfast perseverance looking within, until
Wisdom reveal to us those higher objects of
pursuit and truer attractions which will not
suffer the mind aspiring to them to fall into
dishonour ; but purifying and corroborating as
they draw, will, when at length they are worthily
won, unite with and transmute their worshipper
into that Harmony and Beauty which, in the
dim beholding, he venerated and loved.

> " Begin to-day, nor end till evil sink
> In its due grave ; and if at once we may not
> Declare the greatness of the work we plan
> Be sure at least that ever in our mind
> It stand complete before us, as a dome
> Of light beyond this gloom, a house of stars,
> Encompassing these dusky tents ; a thing
> Absolute, close to all, though seldom seen,
> Near as our Hearts and perfect as the Heavens ;
> Be this our aim and model, and our Hands
> Shall not wax faint until the work is done."

The Idea of the Good, the Pure, and the True
is the alluring object which we all innerly worship—the progeny of Divine Intellect immortal
and strong—even Moral Beauty which, though
obscurely now, through the mists of sense and

selfishness, ever shines attractively our <u>Polar</u> *our guide*
<u>Star</u> :

> " When from the lips of Truth one mighty breath
> Shall, like a whirlwind scatter in its breeze
> The whole dark pile of human mockeries,
> Then shall the reign of Mind commence on earth
> And starting fresh, as from a second birth,
> Man, in the sunshine of the world's new spring,
> Shall walk transparent like some holy thing."

" Already, see, the *hallowed branches wave !*
Hark ! sounds tumultuous shake the trembling cave !
Far, ye profane ! far off ! with beauteous feet
Bright <u>Phœbus</u> comes, and thunders at the gate ; *Phoebus*
See ! the glad sign the *Delian Palm* hath given ;
Sudden it bends ; and, hovering in the Heaven,
Soft sings the swan with melody divine :
BURST OPE, YE BARS ! YE GATES, YOUR HEADS DECLINE !
DECLINE YOUR HEADS ! YE SACRED DOORS EXPAND !
HE COMES ! THE GOD OF LIGHT ! THE GOD'S AT HAND !
Begin the song ; and tread the sacred ground
In mystic dance symphonious to the sound.
Begin, young men ! <u>Apollo's eyes</u> endure
None but the good, the perfect, and the pure,
<u>Who view the God are great,</u> but abject they
From whom he turns his favouring eyes away ;
All piercing God ! in every place confess'd,
We will prepare, behold thee, and be bless'd ;
He comes, young men ! nor silent should ye stand
With harp or feet, when PHŒBUS is at HAND."

Now let us chaunt our breviary,
And show our friends our aviary,
Is not this good behaviour, eh ?

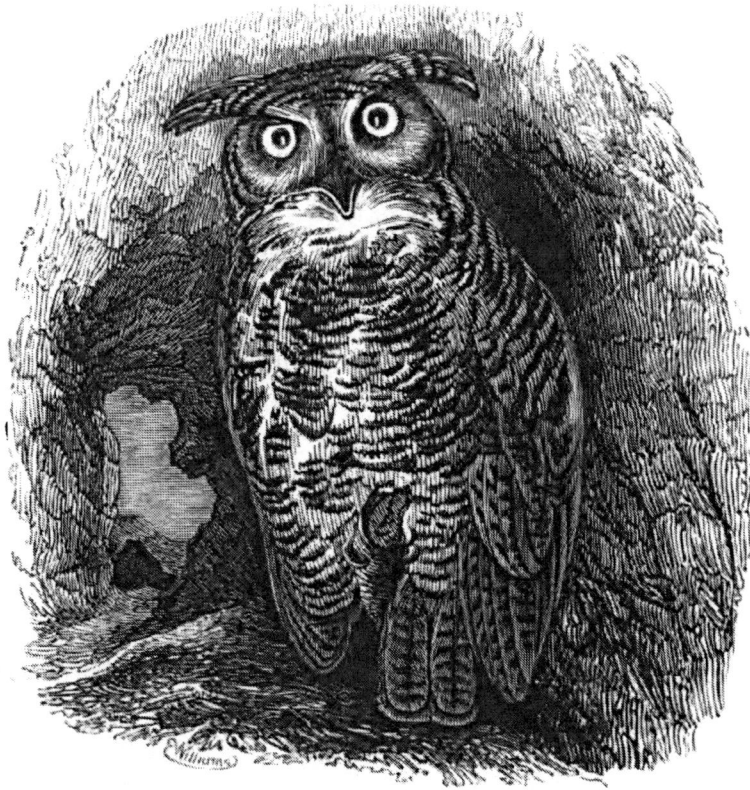

Bird of the night ! Minerva bade thee fly
  Only at length, when dusky evening fades,
That then to heights of metaphor thine eye
  Might dart, or dive in allegory's shades :

To know, and with thy knowledge be discreet,
  Close with the many, freely with the wise
To hold communion, still to keep thy seat,
  When birds of lighter feather think to rise.

Quick, with the lightening fire she caught from Jove,
  High Pallas saw thee, not in form alone,
But thy wrapt mind, life's common place above,
  She mark'd, adopted, claim'd thee for her own.

Gave thee life's best, first, last, essential boon,
  Clear, as the northern lights in ether play,
From her own forehead, as the nightly moon
  Wears the calm reflex of the solar ray.

The sister Muses, singly floating by,
  Pausing in reverence at her behest,
Pour'd spirit on thy sense, entranced thine eye,
  And in the world's oblivion gave thee rest :
Taught thee how high Olympus was not all
  A baseless fable, feigned, and false, and far ;
Unfolded Chaos to thee, and the fall
  Of proud Prometheus, and the Titan war ;

Young conquering Bacchus, not the reeling clown,
  The wine-drunk God to sensual mortal sense,
But the flush'd Hero worthy of his crown,
  The guerdon gained from Heaven's Omnipotence.

Taught thee, how feathered Mercury doth glide
  Invisible on earth, and rise sublime,
Lifting dull sense through Heaven's high portal wide,
  Where living mortal never hoped to climb.

Not wooden Hermes with the *timber toe*,
  Nor Vatican Apollo though he be,
Nor Vulcan with the vulgar fire below,
  Nor Venus from Apelles' hand just free.

Unveiled the Eleusinian mystic rite,
  Sad Ceres, and the ravish'd Proserpine,
Hades, and Styx, and Erebus, and night,
  Nox, O Noctua ! clear as day was thine.

Glorious Apollo, and the Python slain
  By his bright arm, and virtue's deadlier hate,
Old Saturn in his golden youth again,
  On food like this she bade thee ruminate.

And thou wilt still feed on, and drink thy fill,
  Through musing generations yet unborn,
Drink Wisdom from the pure Parnassian rill,
  And ruminate on Amalthæa's horn.

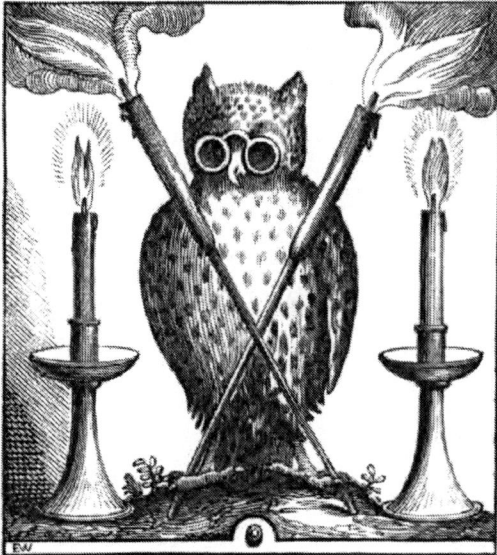

Blind world! seems not this owl a type of thee?
All light of learning darkness to the masses?
Look! of what use for wisdom are the glasses,
The blazing candles and the torches?
Alas! the broad light only scorches;
THE ANIMAL WON'T SEE.

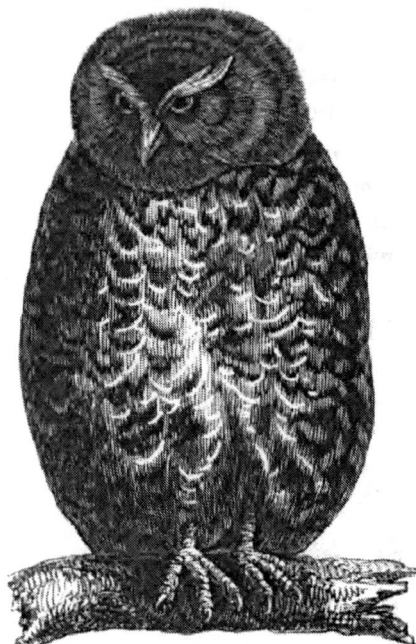

There, still she sits in emblematic guise,
The yet unsolved enigma of the wise ;
All blind without (gainsay it not despite
Of high Minerva) all within is light :
Speak, sacred bird, give utterance divine
To those dark syllables, that all combine,
" Man know thyself!" thou needst nought else to know
For bliss above, and happiness below,
For joy, and health, and peace, or if for gold
Thy thirst, and power, I promise power and gold.
Know but thyself! within, within thou'lt find
The pure light, outwardly like me be blind !
These three short words, all blank to learning's scowl,
And scoffing, loud, loud ! louder, speak, my Owl.

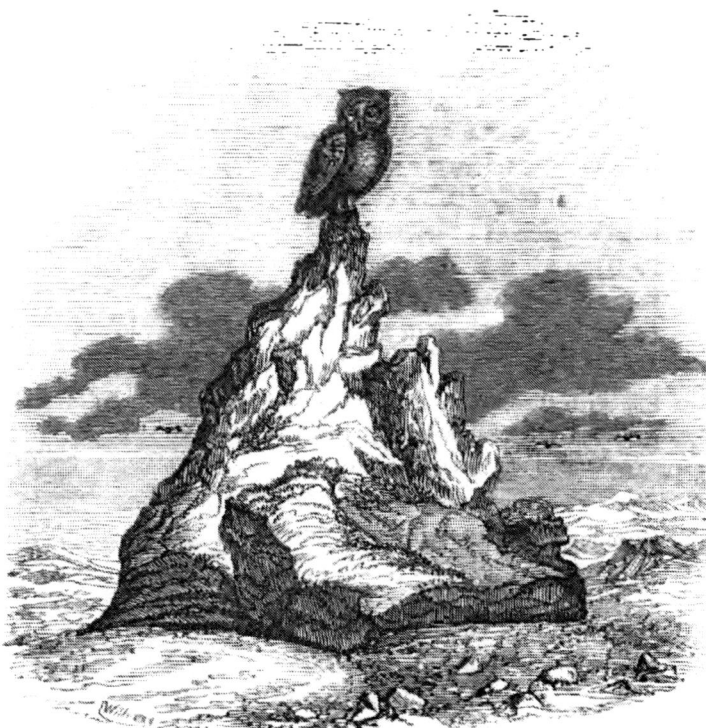

Thou musing, moping, melancholy bird,
What genius drew thee? what ambition stirr'd?
How hast thou climb'd, or flapp'd thy stealthy wing
To heights like these, where songsters cease to sing?
And there thou sit'st exposed, a joyless thing.
Thou darkness visible, in light's own rays,
Of all that fly the mockery and the maze.
Thou would'st not climb, but in thy humbler sphere
Thou wert not happy, and what art thou here?
Wouldst thou aspire thus bodily to stray,

F 2

High as the Polar star or milky way?
In this empyreal ether to presume
Thou art too earthy, and too gross thy plume;
Too dull on earth, high Heaven to explore,
Where Jove's own eagle only dare to soar.
To thee what's nectar? what's ambrosian fare?
All here to thee is thin and empty air;
What's Helicon to thee, and what art thou
To Helicon? look down, thou hast enow
Below to brood on, thick and murky clump
Of frill and feather, still to keep thee plump.
All powerless here, and faint be thy sojourn.
For earth thou art, to earth thou shalt return.
Athenian spirit! light with wisdom's glow,
After life's long ordeal past below,
Freed from thy bonds, thou well may'st here aspire
Once more to rise, and bear Athenian fire.

With drooping wing, and silent as the snow,
In eddying whirl she swoops again below;
And there to mock, soliloquize and grieve,
All day she sits from morn till dewy eve;
Misprized in Heaven, and understood by few
On earth, owls like herself, to whit to whoo!
Seems haunting this vain, busy, trifling ground
Only to hoot, and still to hoot on all around!
And thus a fellow bird, that ne'er has sung
Till now, interprets close thy unknown tongue:

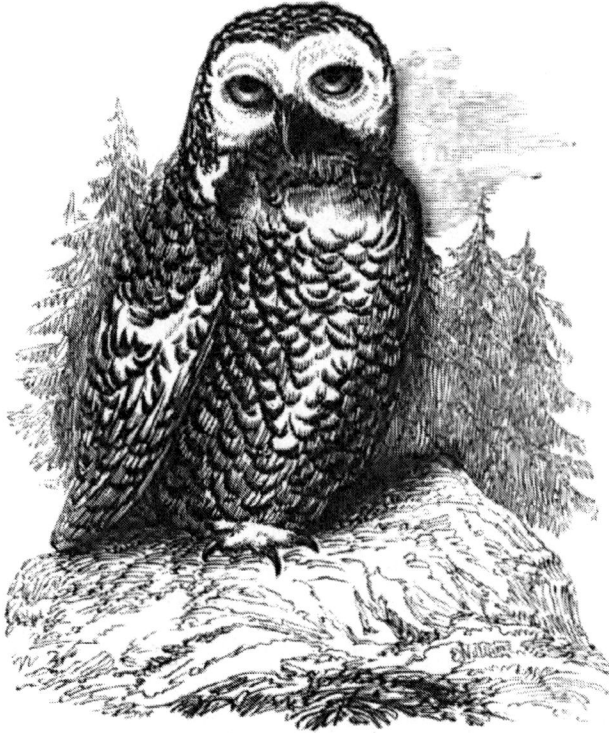

Thou owe'st the penance of thy birth, like all
Gross body ever, ever doom'd to fall,
The forfeit and the pledge of fealty, still
Which all flesh pays before the Sovereign Will ;
But genial spirit, free as vital air,
Soars high and boundless over sense, and dare
All loose from body, lift the immortal soul
From the snake's coil, to join the perfect whole,
With the new light confirm the High Decree.
" THOU SHALT, SHALT HAVE NO OTHER GODS BUT ME."

The subsequent pages are addressed to those
who, not only having seen, are already believers
in Magnetism, but especially to those believers
who *experiencing* the wonders of the trance, and
with minds starting as it were from slumber at
that morning light, have been awakened and
aroused from the long lethargy of ages: from
darkness, and from dreams, and from delusions;
to wonder and to pause, and meditate: to stir
new energies within them, to hail a new existence, to see all glorious day brightening before
them, to beat well without the expansive fields
of eastern lore, to trace the modern specula-
tions, to read, hear, and see, and to shut every
sense and look within.

And having raised the mind by deep soliloquy
and meditation high into the intellectual spheres,
and (if worthy) catching holy light, with new
born awe and reverence have bowed, and from
mercy drawn the inspiration, worshipping that
shrine of which belike they had scant knowledge
heretofore. Some such (many may they be!)
there are, and on them now we strike the deep
responding chords.

My wish and hope are to awaken the public
mind up to a higher faith, a holier view of Magnetism, to approach it reverentially as the wise
and good of old; with pure hearts and suppli-

cating hands, " Not my will, O Lord! but thine
be done:" to feel that there we leave the worldly
dust and mire to tread on holier ground. "Lord,
prosper thou the work of our hands upon us,
O! prosper thou our handy work." " The wind
bloweth where it listeth," it strengtheneth and
refresheth the humble and true-hearted.

Further to introduce the subject with authority from the sacred volume, let me beg leave
here to make some short significant extracts
from the book of Psalms, though from the beginning to the end it is all edifying and illustrative. Has not God's anointed chosen servant
David thus in rapture chanted? and have not
we too with devotion joined in chorus, and yet
happier still have we too caught the inspiration?

" O sing unto the Lord a new song, for he
hath done marvellous things.

" We have heard with our ears, O God! our
fathers have told us the noble works that thou
didst in their days, in the times of old.

" There is sprung up a Light for the righteous,
and joyful gladness for such as are true-hearted.

". Thou hast shewed thy people hard things,
thou hast made us to drink the wine of astonish-
ment.

" Thou hast given a banner to them that fear thee, that it may be displayed because of the truth.

" An unwise man doth not well consider this, and a fool doth not understand it.

" Who shall ascend into the hill of the Lord, and who shall stand in his holy place ?

" He that hath clean hands, and a pure heart, who hath not lift up his soul unto vanity, nor sworn deceitfully.

" He shall receive the blessing from the Lord, and righteousness from the God of his salvation.

" The secret of the Lord is among them, that fear him, and he will show them his covenant.

" I will wash my hands in innocency, O Lord, and so will I go to the altar.

" The Lord my God shall make my darkness to be light.

" To see thy power and thy glory, so as I have seen thee in the sanctuary.

" Thus will I bless thee while I live, I will lift up my hands in thy name.

" And the glorious Majesty of the Lord our God be upon us, and establish thou the work of our hands upon us; yea the work of our hands establish thou it.

" Praise God in the sanctuary, praise him in the firmament of his power.

" Lift up your hands in the sanctuary, and praise the Lord with a mighty hand and an outstretched arm.

" Lord! what is man that thou art mindful of him, and the son of man that thou visitest him ?

" Whoso is wise will ponder these things, and they shall understand the loving kindness of the Lord.

" I have said that ye are gods, and ye are all the children of the Most High.

" But ye shall die like men."

The scriptural extracts that will next be offered, as bearing on this subject, are taken from Solomon and the inspired Isaiah, to them wishing as much as possible to confine myself; the field would be too wide and the receptive knowledge required would be too ample to allow of taking at present a wider range; much self-mistrust and prudence as regards others stay the pen, and with the great masters Isaiah, and with Solomon about to speak, it behoves the scholar to be silent. Well have they spoken for themselves, and now may many eyes and ears be opened to their revealments ; that what we all before have read devotionally, we may now receive with enlightenment ; that we may read, mark, learn, and inwardly digest their time surviving, hallowed words and sacred parables ; that we may embrace and ever hold fast the blessed hope of everlasting life as given us in our Saviour Jesus Christ.

ISAIAH.

" I have long time holden my peace, I have been still and refrained myself.

" Hear, ye deaf, and look, ye blind, that ye may see.

" Seek ye out the book of the Lord, and read.

" Behold, the former things are come to pass, and new things do I declare ; before they spring forth, I tell you of them.

" Let all the nations be gathered together, and let the people be assembled, who among them can declare this, and show us former things ?

" Let them bring forth their witnesses, that they may be justified ; or let them hear, and say, it is truth.

" Bring forth the blind people that have eyes, and the deaf that have ears.

" Who is blind but my servant, or deaf as my messenger that I sent? Who is blind as he that is perfect, and blind as the Lord's servant?

Seeing many things, but thou observest not, opening the ears, but he heareth not.

" Who among you will give ear to this? Who will hearken and hear for the time to come?

" I have not spoken in secret, in a dark place of the earth.

" Look unto me and be saved, all ye ends of the earth.

" Wo unto them that call evil good, and good evil, that put darkness for light, and light for darkness, that are wise in their own eyes, and prudent in their own sight.

" The people that walked in darkness have seen a great light, they that dwell in the land of the shadow of death, upon them hath the light shined.

" For all this his anger is not turned away, but his hand is stretched out still.

" For the earth shall be full of the knowledge of the Lord, as the waters cover the sea.

" In that day shall a man look to his Maker, and his eyes shall have respect to the Holy One of Israel.

" And the key of the house of David will I lay upon his shoulder, so he shall open and none shall shut, and he shall shut, and none shall open.

" Lord! when thy hand is lifted up, they will not see.

" Thou hast wrought all thy work in us.

" Whom shall he teach knowledge, and whom shall he make to understand doctrine?

" Them that are weaned from the milk, and drawn from the breasts.

" For precept must be upon precept, precept upon precept, line upon line, line upon line, here a little, and there a little, for with stammering lips and another tongue will he speak to his people.

" To whom he said, this is the rest wherewith ye may cause the weary to rest, and this is the refreshing.

" Yet they would not hear.

" This also cometh from the Lord of Hosts, which is wonderful in counsel, and excellent in working.

" And thou shalt be brought down, and shalt speak out of the ground, and thy voice shall be low out of the dust, and thy voice shall be as one that hath a familiar spirit, out of the ground, and thy speech shall whisper out of the dust.

Moreover the multitude of thy strangers shall be like small dust;

" Stay yourselves and wonder, cry ye out and cry, they are drunken, but not with wine, they stagger, but not with strong drink.

" For the Lord hath poured out upon you the spirit of deep sleep, and hath closed your eyes; the prophets and your rulers, the seers hath he covered.

" And the vision of all is become unto you as the words of a book that is sealed, which men deliver to one that is learned, saying, read this I pray thee, and he saith, I cannot for it is sealed.

And the book is delivered to him, that is not learned, saying, read this I pray thee, and he saith, I am not learned.

" Therefore the Lord said; forasmuch as this people draw near me with their mouth, and with their lips do honour me, but have removed their heart far from me, and their fear towards me is taught by the precept of men.

" Therefore behold I will proceed to do a marvellous work amongst this people, even a marvellous work and a wonder; for the wisdom of their wise men shall perish, and the understanding of their prudent men shall be hid.

" Wo unto them that seek deep to hide their

counsel from the Lord, and their works are in
the dark, and they say, who seeth us, and who
knoweth us.

"And in that day shall the deaf hear the
words of the book, and the eyes of the blind
shall see out of obscurity and out of darkness.

"The meek also shall increase their joy in the
Lord, and the poor among men shall rejoice in
the Holy One of Israel.

"They that have erred in spirit shall come to
understanding, and they that murmured shall
learn doctrine.

"Now go write it before them in a table, and
note it in a book, that it may be for the time to
come, for ever and for ever.

"That this is a rebellious people, lying children, children that will not hear the law of the
Lord.

"Which say to the seers, see not, and to the
prophets, prophecy not unto us right things,
speak unto us smooth things, prophecy de-
ceits.

"Get you out of the way, turn aside out of
the path : cause the Holy One of Israel to cease
from before us.

"Wherefore thus saith the Holy One of
Israel, because ye despise this word, and

trust in oppression and perverseness, and stay thereon ;

" One thousand shall flee at the rebuke of one, at the rebuke of five shall ye flee.

" He shall lift up his staff against thee after the manner of Egypt.

" Now the Egyptians are men and not God, and their horses are flesh and not spirit ; when the Lord shall stretch out his hand, both he that helpeth shall fall, and he that is holpen shall fall down, and they shall all fail together.

" But the liberal deviseth liberal things, and by liberal things shall he stand.

" Now will I rise, saith the Lord, now will I be exalted, now will I lift up myself ;

" Fear not, for I am with thee, be not dismayed, for I am thy God, I will strengthen thee, yea I will help thee, yea I will uphold thee with the right hand of my righteousness.

" For I the Lord thy God will hold thy right hand, saying unto thee, fear not, for I will help thee.

" And the eyes of them that see shall not be dim, and the ears of them that hear shall hearken :

" The heart also of the rash shall understand knowledge.

" And the tongue of the stammerer shall be ready to speak plainly.

" One shall say, I am the Lord's, and another shall call himself by the name of Jacob, and another shall subscribe himself with his hand unto the Lord, and surname himself with the name of Jacob.

" Thus saith the Lord, the King of Israel, and his Redeemer, the Lord of Hosts, I am the first, and I am the last, and besides me there is no God, and who as I shall declare it and set it in order for me since I appointed the ancient people ? And the things that are coming shall come.

" That unto me every knee shall bow, every tongue shall swear.

" For I am God, declaring the end from the beginning, and from the ancient times the things that are not yet done.

" Saying my counsel shall stand, and I will do all my pleasure.

" Therefore my people have gone into captivity, because they have no knowledge.

" Strengthen ye the weak hands and confirm the feeble knees ; say to them that are of a fearful heart, be strong fear not.

" Behold your God, with a recompense, will come and save you.

"Then the eyes of the blind shall be opened, and the ears of the deaf shall be unstopped.

"Then shall the lame man leap up as an hart, and the tongue of the dumb sing.

"Who is he among you that feareth the Lord, that obeyeth the voice of his servant, that walketh in darkness and hath no light?

"Let him trust in the name of the Lord, and stay upon his God.

"Behold, all ye that kindle a fire, that compass yourselves about with sparks, walk in the light of your fire, and in the sparks that ye have kindled;

"This shall ye have of mine hands, ye shall lie down in sorrow.

"Hearken unto me, ye that follow after right courses, ye that seek the Lord;

"Look unto the rock whence ye are hewn, and to the hole of the pit, whence ye are digged.

"I even I am he that comforteth you. Who art thou that thou shouldst be afraid of a man that shall die, and of the son of man which shall be made as grass?

"And forgettest the Lord thy Maker, that hath stretched forth the heavens, and laid the foundations of the earth.

"How beautiful upon the mountains are the

feet of him that bringeth good tidings of good; that publisheth salvation, that saith unto Zion, thy Lord reigneth.

"The Lord hath made bare his holy arm in the eyes of all nations, and all the ends of the earth shall see the salvation of our God.

"So shall he sprinkle many nations, the kings shall shut their mouths at him, for that which had not been told them shall they see, and that which they had not heard shall they consider.

"Who hath believed our report, and to whom is the arm of the Lord revealed?

"Wherefore do ye spend money for that which is not bread, and your labour for that which satisfieth not?

"Hearken diligently unto me, and eat ye that which is good.

"Thus saith the Lord, keep ye judgment, and do justice, for my salvation is near to come, and my righteousness to be revealed.

"His watchmen are blind, they are all dumb dogs, they cannot bark, lying down, loving to slumber;

"Yea they are all greedy dogs, which can never have enough, and they are shepherds that cannot understand.

"They all look to their own way, every one to his gain from his quarter.

" Associate yourselves, O ye people! and ye shall be broken in pieces.

"Take counsel together, and it shall come to nought; speak the word, and it shall not stand;

" For God is with us.

" For the Lord spake thus unto me with a strong hand, and instructed me, that I should not walk in the way of this people.

" Wherefore have we fasted? say they! and thou seest not, wherefore have we afflicted our souls, and thou takest no knowledge?

" Behold, in the day of your fast, you find pleasure, and exact all your labours.

" Behold ye fast for strife and debate, and to smite with the fist of wickedness.

" Ye shall not fast as ye do this day to make your voice be heard on high.

"Is it for such a fast that I have chosen a day for a man to afflict his soul?

" Is it to bow down his head as a bulrush, and to spread sackcloth and ashes under him? Wilt thou call this a fast, and an acceptable day to the Lord?

" Is not this the fast that I have chosen?

" To loose the bands of wickedness? To undo the heavy burden, and to let the oppressed go free, and that ye break every yoke?

G 2

"Is it not to deal thy bread to the hungry, and that thou bring the poor that are captive to thy house ?

"When thou seest the naked that thou cover him, and that thou hide not thyself from thine own flesh ?

"Then shall thy light break forth as the morning, and thine health shall spring forth speedily :

"And thy righteousness shall go before thee, the glory of the Lord shall be thy reward.

"Then shalt thou call, and the Lord shall answer ; thou shalt cry, and he shall say, here I am ! If thou take away from the midst of thee the yoke, the putting forth of the finger, and speaking vanity :

"And if thou draw out thy soul to the hungry, and satisfy the afflicted soul ;

"Then shall thy light rise in obscurity, and thy darkness be as the noon-day.

"And the Lord shall guide thee continually, and satisfy thy soul in drought, and make fat thy bones, and thou shalt be like a watered garden, and like a spring of water, whose waters fail not.

"And if thou turn away thy foot from the sabbath, from doing thy pleasure on my holy day, and call the sabbath a delight, the holy of the Lord, honourable, and shall honour him, not doing thine own ways, nor speaking thine own words :

" Then shalt thou delight thyself in the Lord, and I will cause thee to ride upon the high places of the earth, and feed thee with the heritage of Jacob thy father.

" For the mouth of the Lord hath spoken it.

" Behold the Lord's hand is not shortened, that it cannot save, neither is his ear heavy that it cannot hear.

" But your iniquities have separated between you and your God, and your sins have hid his face from you, that he will not hear.

" Therefore is judgment far from us, neither doth justice overtake us :

" We wait for light, but behold obscurity, for brightness, but we walk in darkness ;

" We grope as if we had no eyes, we stumble at noon-day as in the night.

" We look for judgment, but there is none ; for salvation, but it is far from us.

" For our transgressions are multiplied before thee, and our sins testify against us, for our transgressions are with us, and as for our iniquities, we know them.

" And judgment is turned away backward,

and justice standeth afar off, for truth is fallen in the streets, and equity cannot enter.

"Yea, truth faileth, and he that departeth from evil, maketh himself a prey.

"And the Lord saw it, and it displeased him that there was no judgment.

"And he saw that there was no man, and wondered that there was no intercessor.

"Therefore his arm brought salvation unto him, and his righteousness it sustained him.

"For he put on righteousness as a breast-plate, and an helmet of salvation upon his head : and he put on the garments of vengeance for clothing, and was clad with zeal as a cloak.

"Arise, shine, for thy light is come, and the glory of the Lord is risen upon thee.

"For behold, the darkness shall cover the earth, and gross darkness the people ; but the Lord shall arise upon thee, and his glory shall be seen upon thee.

"And the Gentiles shall come to thy light, and kings to the brightness of thy rising.

"The sun shall be no more thy light by day, neither for brightness shall the moon give light unto thee, but the Lord shall be unto thee an everlasting light, and thy God thy glory.

" Thy sun shall no more go down, neither shall thy moon withdraw itself.

" For the Lord shall be thine everlasting light, and the days of thy mourning 'shall be ended.

" The spirit of the Lord is upon me, because the Lord hath anointed me to preach good tidings unto the meek, he hath sent me to bind up the broken-hearted, to proclaim liberty to the captives, and the opening of the prison to them that are bound.

" To proclaim the acceptable year of the Lord, and the day of vengeance of our God.

" To comfort all that mourn, to give them beauty for ashes, the oil of joy for mourning, the garment of praise for the spirit of heaviness :

" That they might be called trees of righteousness, the planting of the Lord.

PROVERBS.

" Happy is the man that findeth wisdom, and the man that getteth understanding.

" Length of days is in her right hand, and in her left hand riches and honour.

" She is a tree of life to them that lay hold upon her, and happy is every one that retaineth her.

"Withhold not good from them to whom it is due, when it is in the power of thine hand to do it.

"I, wisdom, dwell with prudence, and find out knowledge of witty inventions.

"The fear of the Lord is the beginning of wisdom, and the knowledge of the Holy One is understanding.

"The fear of the Lord is the beginning of knowledge, but fools despise wisdom and instruction.

"My son, hear the instruction of thy father, and forsake not the law of thy mother.

"For they shall be an ornament of grace unto thine head, and chains about thy neck.

"Let thine eyes look right on, and let thine eyelids look straight before thee;

"To understand a proverb, and the interpretation, the words of the wise, and their dark sayings.

"For the spirit of the Lord filleth the world, and that which containeth all things hath knowledge of the voice.

"Seek not death in the error of your life, and pull not upon yourselves destruction with the works of your hands.

"How long, ye simple ones, will ye love sim-

plicity, and the scorners delight in their scorn-
ing, and fools hate knowledge?

" I have stretched out my hand, and no man
regarded, for they that hated knowledge, and did
not choose the fear of the Lord, they would
none of my counsel, they despised all my re-
proof.

" If thou criest after knowledge, and liftest up
thy voice for understanding;

" If thou seekest for her as silver, and search-
est for her as for hid treasures,

" Then shalt thou understand the fear of the
Lord, and find the knowledge of God;

" For the Lord giveth wisdom, out of his
mouth cometh understanding.

" His secret is with the righteous.

" Get wisdom, get understanding, forget it
not, neither decline from the words of my
mouth.

" Wisdom is the principal thing, therefore get
wisdom, and with all thy getting get understanding.

" She shall give to thy head a crown of
grace, a crown of glory shall she deliver unto
thee.

" Take fast hold of instruction, let her not go,
keep her, for she is thy life.

"My son, forget not my law, let thine heart keep my commandments.

"For length of days, and long life, and peace shall they add to thee.

"Be not wise in thine own eyes, fear the Lord, and depart from evil.

"A scorner seeketh wisdom, and findeth it not, but knowledge is easy to him that understandeth.

"The spirit of man is the candle of the Lord, searching all the inward parts of his belly.

"A false balance is an abomination to the Lord, but a just weight is his delight.

"Who hath ascended up into heaven, or descended?

"Who hath gathered the wind in his fists?

"Who hath bound the waters in a garment?

"Who hath established all the ends of the earth, what is his name, and what is his son's name, if thou canst tell?

WISDOM OF SOLOMON.

"As for wisdom, what she is, and how she came up, I will tell you, and will not hide mysteries from you;

"But will seek her out from the beginning of

her nativity, and bring the knowledge of her unto light, and will not pass over the truth.

" For the true beginning of her is the desire of discipline, and the care of discipline is love.

" Whoso seeketh her early shall have no great travel, for he shall find her sitting at his doors.

"Receive therefore instruction through my words, and it shall do you good.

" I prayed, and understanding was given me, I called upon God, and the spirit of wisdom came to me.

" I preferred her before sceptres and thrones, and esteemed riches nothing in comparison of her.

" I loved her above health and beauty, and chose to have her instead of light.

" For the light that cometh from her never goeth out.

"I learned diligently, and do communicate her liberally.

" I do not hide her riches.

" Wisdom opened the mouth of the dumb, and made the tongues of them that cannot speak eloquent.

" She prospered their works in the hands of the holy prophet.

"It was neither herb nor mollifying plaister that restored them to health ;

"But thy word, O Lord, which healeth all things, for thine incorruptible spirit is in all things.

"And to know thy power is the root of immortality.

"God hath granted me to speak as I would, and to conceive as is meet for the things that are given me, because it is He that leadeth unto wisdom and directeth the wise.

"For in his hand are both we and our words.

"All wisdom, also, and knowledge of workmanship ;

"For he hath given me certain knowledge of the things that are, namely, to know how the world was made, and the operation of the elements,

"The beginning, ending, and midst of the times, the alterations of the turning of the sun, and the change of seasons,

"The circuits of years, and the position of the stars ;

"The natures of living creatures, and the furies of wild beasts, the violence of winds, and the reasonings of men ; the diversities of plants, and the virtues of roots ;

" And all such things as are either secret or manifest, them I know.

" For wisdom which is the worker of all things taught me, for in her is an understanding spirit, holy, one only, manifold, subtile, lively, clear, undefiled, plain ;

" Not subject to hurt, loving the thing that is good, quick, which cannot be letted, ready to do good ;

" Kind to man, steadfast, sure, free from care, having all power, overseeing all things, and going through all understanding, pure and most subtile spirit.

"For wisdom is more moving than any motion, she passeth and goeth through all things by reason of her pureness.

" For she is the breath of the power of God, and a pure influence flowing from the power of the Almighty ; therefore can no undefiled thing fall into her.

" For she is the brightness of the everlasting light, the unspotted mirror of the power of God, and the image of his goodness.

" And being but one, she can do all things ;

" And remaining in herself, she maketh all things new, and in all ages entering into holy souls, she maketh them friends of God and prophets.

" For God loveth none, but him that dwelleth with wisdom.

" For she is more beautiful than the sun.

" And above all the order of stars; being compared with the light, she is found before it;

" For after this cometh night, but vice shall not prevail against wisdom.

" Wisdom reacheth from one to another, mightily, and sweetly doth she order all things.

" I loved her, and sought her out from my youth, I desired to make her my spouse.

" And I was a lover of her beauty.

" In that she is conversant with God, she magnifyeth her nobility; yea, the Lord of all things himself loved her.

" For she is privy to the mysteries of the knowledge of God, and lover of his works.

" If riches be a possession to be desired in this life, what is richer than wisdom, that worketh all things?

" And if prudence work, who of all that are, is a more cunning workman than she?

" And if a man love righteousness, her labours are virtues, for she teacheth temperance and prudence, justice, and fortitude, which are such things as men can have nothing more profitable in their life.

" If a man desire much experience, she knoweth things of old, and conjectureth aright what is to come; she knoweth the subtleties of speeches, and can expound dark sentences; she foreseeth signs and wonders, and the events of seasons and times.

" Therefore I purposed to take her to me to live with me, knowing that she would be a counsellor of good things, and a comfort in cares and grief.

" For her sake I shall have an estimation among the multitude, and honour with the elders though I be young.

" I shall be found of a quick conceit in judgment, and shall be admired in the sight of great men.

" When I hold my tongue, they shall bide my leisure, and when I speak they shall give good ear unto me.

" If I talk much they shall lay their hands upon their mouth.

" Moreover, by the means of her, I shall obtain immortality, and leave behind me an everlasting memorial to them that come after me.

" Horrible tyrants shall be afraid, when they do but hear me, and I shall be found good among the multitude, and valiant in war.

" After I am come into mine house, I will repose myself with her ; for her conversation hath no bitterness, and to live with her hath no sorrow, but mirth and joy.

"Now when I considered these things in myself, and pondered them in mine heart, how that to be allied unto wisdom is immortality,

"And great pleasure is it to have her friendship, and in the works of her hands are infinite riches, and in the exercise of conference with her, prudence, and in talking with her a good report;

"I went about seeking how to take her to me,

"For I was a witty child, and had a good spirit.

"Yea, rather being good, I came into a body undefiled.

"Nevertheless, when I perceived that I could not otherwise obtain her, except God gave her to me (and that was a point of wisdom also to know whose gift she was), I prayed unto the Lord, and besought him, and with my whole heart I said :

"O God of my fathers and Lord of mercy, who hast made all things with thy Word, and ordained man through thy wisdom, that he should have dominion over the creatures which thou hast made,

" And order the world according to equity and righteousness, and execute judgments with an upright heart,

" Give me wisdom, that sitteth by thy throne, and reject me not from among thy children ;

" For I thy servant and son of thine hand-maid, am a feeble person and of a short time, and too young for the understanding of judgment and laws.

" For though a man be never so perfect among the children of men, yet if thy wisdom be not with him, he shall be nothing regarded.

" Thou hast chosen me to be a king of thy people, and a judge of thy sons and daughters,

" Thou hast commanded me to build a temple upon thy holy mount, and an altar in the city wherein thou dwellest,

" A resemblance of the holy tabernacle which thou hast prepared from the beginning.

" And wisdom was with thee, which knoweth thy works, and was present when thou madest the world, and knew what was acceptable in thy sight, and right in thy commandments.

" O ! send her out of thy holy heavens, and from the throne of thy glory, that being present

H

she may labour with me, that I may know what is pleasing unto thee.

"For she knoweth and understandeth all things, and she shall lead me soberly in my doings, and preserve me in her power.

"So shall my works be acceptable, and then shall I judge thy people righteously,

"And be'worthy to sit in my father's seat.

"For what man is he that can know the counsel of God? Or who can think what the will of the Lord is?

"For the thoughts of mortal men are miserable, and our desires are but uncertain.

"For the corruptible body presseth down the soul, and the earthy tabernacle weigheth down the mind that museth upon many things.

"And hardly do we guess aright of things that are upon earth, and with labour do we find the things that are before us;

"But the things that are in heaven, who hath searched out?

"And thy counsel, who hath known? Except thou give wisdom, and send thy holy spirit from above.

"For so the ways of them which lived on the earth were reformed, and men were taught the things that are pleasing unto thee;

"And were saved through wisdom.

" For God created man to be immortal, and made him to be an image of his own eternity.

ECCLESIASTICUS.

" Who shall set a watch before my mouth, and a seal of wisdom upon my lips, that I fall not suddenly by them, and that my tongue destroy me not?

" Be not curious in unnecessary matters, for more things are shewed unto thee than men understand.

" But what is commanded thee, think thereupon with reverence, for it is not needful for thee to see with thine eyes the things that are in secret.

" Many are in high places and of renown, but mysteries are revealed unto the meek.

" Draw near unto me, you unlearned, and dwell in the house of learning.

" Wherefore are ye slow, and what say you of these things, seeing your souls are very thirsty.

" Wisdom hath been created before all things, and the understanding of prudence from everlasting.

"The word of God most high is the foundation of wisdom.

"She is with all flesh according to his gift, and he hath given her to them that love him. ·

"Search and seek, and she shall be made known unto thee, and when thou hast got hold of her, let her not go.

"I am the mother of fair love, and fear, and knowledge, and holy hope; I therefore being eternal am given to all my children which are named of Him.

"Come unto me all ye that be desirous of me, and fill yourselves with my fruits.

"He that obeyeth me shall never be confounded, and they that work by me shall not do amiss.

"The wisdom of a learned man cometh by opportunity of leisure, and he that hath little business shall become wise.

"How can he get wisdom that holdeth the plough, and that glorieth in the goad? That driveth oxen, and is occupied in their labours, whose talk is of bullocks?

"But he that giveth his mind to the law of the Most High, and is occupied in the meditation thereof, will seek out the wisdom of all the ancient, and be occupied in prophecies.

"He will keep the sayings of renowned men, and where subtle parables are, he will be there also;

"He will seek out the secrets of grave sentences, and be conversant in dark parables.

"He will give his heart to resort early to the Lord that made him, and will pray before the Most High, and will open his mouth in prayer, and make supplication for his sins.

"When the great Lord will, he shall be filled with the spirit of understanding, he shall pour out wise sentences, and give thanks to the Lord in prayer.

"He shall direct his counsel and knowledge, and in his secrets shall he meditate.

"He shall shew forth that which he hath learned, and shall glory in the law of the covenant of the Lord.

"Yet have I more to say which I have thought upon, for I am filled as the moon at the full.

"My son, if thou come to serve the Lord, prepare thy soul for temptation.

"Turn not away thine eyes from the needy, and give him none occasion to curse thee;

"For, if he curse thee in the bitterness of his soul, his prayer shall be heard of Him that made him.

" I will yet pour out doctrine, and leave it to all ages for ever.

" Behold, I have not laboured for myself only, but for all them that seek wisdom.

" The love of the Lord passeth all things for illumination ; faith is the beginning of cleaving unto him.

" Have mercy upon us, O Lord God of all! and behold us, and send thy fear upon all the nations that seek not after thee.

" Lift up thine hand against the strange nations, and let them see thy power, and let them know thee as we have known thee.

" Shew new signs, and make other strange wonders, glorify thy hand and thy right arm, that they may set forth thy wondrous works.

" Who is as the wise man, and who knoweth the interpretation of a thing ?

" A man's wisdom maketh his face to shine, and the boldness of his face shall be changed.

" He declareth the things that are past, and are to come, and readeth the steps of hidden things.

" No thought escapeth him, neither any word is hidden from him, that a man see, even to a spark.

" All things are double, one against another, he hath established nothing imperfect.

" One thing establisheth the good of another.

" Honour the Physician with the honour due unto him, for the uses which you may have of him, for the Lord hath created him.

" For of the Most High cometh healing, and he shall receive honour of the King.

" The skill of the Physician shall lift up his head, and in the sight of great men he shall be in admiration.

" He hath given men skill, that he might be honoured in his marvellous works.

" There is a time when in their hands there is a good success.

" For they also shall pray unto the Lord that he would prosper that which they give for ease, and remedy to prolong life.

" There be yet hid greater things than these be, for we have seen but a few of his works.

" The light shineth in darkness, and the darkness comprehendeth it not."

Yet more awakening than day's harbinger it shines, this dawn of Universal Light! Who now may stay its brightening career? They cannot if they would, they ought not if they could.

Hence, then, not, " truth *against* the world," but
" truth *for* the world," be our pass-word and
countersign.   And let us not think our bodies
only are to move by rail and steam ; the nobler
spheres of mind, too, are expanding, and she,
too, is starting on her course ; and, as the electric
wire outspeeds her laggart rival by her side, so
far more glorious and above shall intellect surpass it in her new elastic bound to loftier inspirations, even as free thought outstrips the cumbrous body.

Many quiet, still, reflecting minds must certainly ere now have been stirred, raised, and
lightened since first this new leaven of Magnetism has been cast on them ; dull and torpid
verily, has been the stuff and clay whereon it
has fallen, that has not felt its working.

" Caligo hæc ingens, quæ vos cognoscere verum
Posse vetat, tolle hanc, oculi meliora videbunt.
Et quæ nunc bona prima putas, fortasse negabis
Esse bona, et quæ nunc credis mala maxima, forsan
Non mala sunt, dices, pulsis a corde tenebris.
Est acies mentis potior, quæ perspicit intus
Quicquid in abstruso est, quicunque hâc utitur, ille
Verus erit rerum judex, et mira videbit."

The days of ignorance pass on ; for long,
dark ages have we dared to drive forth nature
from her field ; with forks and with staves

have expelled her, but ever rallying, she returns, reclaiming her own rights, and confound-
ing human subtlety and assumption; for her at
length the time of retribution has drawn nigh,
when every coming throe shall bring forth
tidings of revealment.

"Omnia jam fiunt, fieri quæ posse negantur,
　Et nihil est de quo non sit habenda fides."

In fundamental principles, nature has ever
been the same, yesterday, to-day, and to-mor-
row,
"I am what was, and is, and shall be."
But how differently, how vaguely has man
looked her in the face; trusting vainly to his own
senses has he beheld her, for which her spirit
was far too subtle and refined. Truly some few
of finer essence, some aspiring mortals have at
intervals arisen, but their light has still been
darkness to the many; the vulgar herd have
gazed and gaped in wonder, and scarcely con-
ceiving what they saw, and judging of others by
themselves, whatever they saw not, felt not in
their own obtuseness, have been unwilling to
believe from others more gifted or more enlightened than themselves.

" Quàre non mirum est, si nostris credere dictis
Turba nequit, siquidem turbæ crassissima mens est.
Talpa bipes, altâ semper tellure sepultus,
Aspiciens nunquam sublato lumine cælum.

A mystery! a miracle! have they cried, and
been content, when for a moment some great
one, lifting Nature's veil, has disclosed some
flitting feature of her ample face. Fair truth
has often been revealed, but rarely examined,
and never appreciated; and when perchance
man might have caught and worshipped her,
base selfishness has intervened, and cast her
cloud over the tabernacle. But the mighty
magician is gone forth; the fiery pillar is before;
follow! follow where it leads, even though it
draw us (whither assuredly it tends), to truth's
everlasting sanctuary.

Look at the wonderful agent in common with
us all, the wonder-working Will, strong in faith,
the great portentous achiever in times of yore,
drawing the substance of things hoped for, the
evidence of the yet unseen realities of thought,
beyond those bounds that give to airy nothing a
local habitation and a name, *ignota vulgo*, fleet-
ing and viewless as the winds in ordinary life,
but *stuff*, perchance, to work on, could we but
apply the proper press and power.

> " corpus sed carceris instar
> Est animæ, quam dum membrorum viribus arctè
> Implicat, æthereæ mentis suffocat acumen,
> Haud secus ac intus positam vas fictile flammam."

Were we not fallen, or could we still regain the high estate! could we but be lifted over sense, sublimed by yearnings pure and strong to be, what we behold! Subduing, crucifying, subjecting wholly our blind will; merging the individual in the universal; thinking, hoping, believing only in the good, and leaving every earthly, earth-born care and cumbrance behind, to rise and poise in happy equilibrium with the etherial perfect whole.

> " I segreti del ciel sol colui vede,
>   Chi serra gli occhi e crede."
> (Secrets divine he sees, and only he
>   Who shuts his eyes, in perfect faith to see.)

" Whosoever exalteth himself shall be humbled, and he who humbleth himself shall be exalted."

Hath not the plying Charon wafted us, and are we not sojourners in Elysium? And may we not each in his own natural, embryotic, preconceptive sphere, moral, intellectual, or divine, bask in pure sunshine? Or be *secundum artem* borne through this world's varying scene, far and away with sure and prying ken, or view all wide without and deep within the present, past, and future as in a molten glass. The broad land-scape lies before us plain and palpable as, to our open eye, this page we now peruse. Nor is this fancy's dream, or conjured up to serve appliances ; but 'tis the vital truth, approachable, I trust appreciable by many, (mortal though we be), humble and meek, let me insist, and willing to walk into the sanctuary. There, too, shall we learn that best lesson life can teach, sub-dued and suffering faith, bowing to kiss the rod. Deep knowledge of dark self, " to what height thou seest, to that depth fallen !" And lingering, we shall rise from the confessional (but entering albeit in fast and prayer), wiser and better, leaving our dross behind. Thus has the indistinct small light, first in modern times discerned, and first announced by Mesmer, with healing in its train, been gradually nearing and brightening in its course, and has in the intel-lectual horizon already caught the gaze of many ; but verily the many little wot of that on which they gaze.

> " Natus humo despectat humum, et terrestria toto
>   Corde petens, cælo quærere nescit opes :
> Nempe rubo similis, nam cum surrexit in altum
>   Radices summâ fronde recurvat humo."

Steadily, and over all, and through all the

base passions of the worldly blind, the growing
light advances; the watchers heed it not, but
the all-vigilant inner sense that never can be-
tray, has still kept it in the focus of its ardent
ken closely observed and hailed it. Cold
and wary watchers, cry, O tell it not in Gath ¡
but we would bring good tidings to the people.
What vista comes before us ? Is the secret
of all ages, the deep root of fable, the whole
mythological mystery, after the long gradual
sleep and certain death of eighteen centuries,
now to be disinterred? (O hear, ye Archæolo-
gists), shorn of its pagan beams, but still
dazzling in its splendour, in its revealed, intelligible beauty! The gorgeous Pantheon that
at the Saviour's light grew dim, that

> " Saw a brighter sun appear,
> Than its proud dome or borrowed pageantry could bear."

And that, like the baseless fabric of a vision,
vanished, leaving no wreck behind. Are we
to burst through the lava of old time, and
like pale, startled ghosts, to wander once again
among the ruins ? And with the blazing torch,
too, shall we pass and pause, and with new
lore expounding every niche and pedestal,
proclaim new voices from the dead! Such cannot " like a summer's dream pass over us

without our special wonder." When after the
long conflicting ordeal of human passions and
enduring faith, the inner man, a giant re-
freshed, at length walks forth upon this worldly
scene. The royal road is now the public way;
the patriarchal privilege hath descended too on
us, and filmy, fishy scales have fallen from our
eyes. And shall we doubt by journeying thereon we yet may reach at length the Holy City?
And there in unpolluted ether again draw fresh
influence to bestow new blessings; and thus
with palms put forth from inward faith, and
emanating holy air, bring joy, and health, and
peace, whereon they fall, to wipe off every tear
from every eye, to pour essential oil and Gilead's
balm.

Look only back to those not distant days of
simpler, livelier faith, when the royal hand in
pure good will was wont to fall with healing
in its touch. "The quality of mercy is not
strained, it droppeth as the gentle dew from
heaven upon the place beneath; it is twice
blessed; it blesses him that gives and him that
takes, 'tis mightiest in the mightiest, and
becomes the throned monarch better than his
crown." And from our slight experience,
friends, can we not foretaste all this, and more
beyond? May we not lift the inward conscious

eye, and catch the golden cup, and trembling draw and drink in ether the pure draught that yet we symbolize in wine ? Think ye that nectar and ambrosia too, are all such vague and empty words, whereof the worthy have not tasted, known, and felt, and seen ?

> " Ergo felices vivunt, nectarque bibentes
> Ambrosiæ viridi pascuntur gramine, cujus
> Copia magna oritur passim cælestibus arvis.
> Verum hæc non sapiunt vulgo, nec talia vulgus
> Credere vult ; quid tum ? Gemmas ne apponite porcis,
> Credite, vos docti, quibus est meus altior.
> Sed cunctis non nosse datum est mysteria divûm,
> Pauci hæc percipiunt, mundi quibus annuit autor,
> Datque suum, ut possint speculari talia, lumen.
> Quàre danda opera in primis, ut simus ad unguem
> Purgati nitidi, puri, et sine sordibus ullis,
> Veste atrâ exuti, et niveo candore decori."

The lusty pioneers, brave men and true, have nobly led the van ; worthily let us too help to fill the breach that leads to suffering man's redemption.

But here, friends, pausing let us beware we touch on holy land, and if it be your glory still with infidels to battle, and utterly to cast away the works of darkness, in honest, fervent zeal then, put ye on the true armour of light, that so with the invulnerable shield and well attempered arm we may pursue our sure career, conquering,

and to conquer. Ere we rush on, bethink us,
we come not to destroy, be it but ours to save.
And ere we stand dauntless here to wield an
anceps flaming sword, O let us look well around
us and before us, lest we hereafter cast a long-
ing lingering look behind. 'Twere glorious to
behold the forked lightning flash, did we not
dread, awe struck, the rifting thunderbolt;

"O! Man *Divine!* thy strength may be thy bane."

Yea verily, 'tis sacred ground we tread on, as
told us by the wise and gifted seers of old, in
words of holy writ, ambiguous now no more; and
though we would not thus in our dark ignorance
misgive, or deem the sacred veil of that invio-
lable holy temple may by profane Hands be
rent in twain; yet, gazing on the flash, can we
be wholly unappalled?

"But my thoughts are not your thoughts,
neither are my ways your ways, saith the
Lord.

"For as much as the Heavens are higher
than the earth, so are my ways higher than
your ways, and my thoughts than your thoughts.

"This is the purpose that is purposed upon
the whole earth, and this is the hand that is
stretched out upon all the nations.

"For the Lord of Hosts hath purposed, and

who shall disannul it, and his hand is stretched out, and who shall turn it back."—*Isaiah*.

Happy they, who in this world's pilgrimage have by their good genius been directed through the labyrinths of science to the goal of Wisdom, along a flowery beguiling way to the central *arbor vitæ* and the golden fruit!

From this spreading tree of knowledge already has sprung up a new and mighty branch, the towering limb of Phreno-magnetism in the wide watery waste of metaphysics.

Gall

Here let us briefly pause then to admire how Gall, the great master, first struck these sources of intellect with his divining rod; when Mesmer's wand came following close behind; but not till lately have they worked in concert; their magic power combined would seem to form a talisman most potent, evocating fresh spirits of light up from the vasty deep; and if they come when we do call, O! ponder on their sybilline responses.

Bethink us still, 'tis sacred ground we tread on, and the Pythia shakes her laurel. Proclaim to man what man is!

" Lord, what is man that thou art mindful of

him, and the son of man that thou so regardest him?"

Slowly, reverently and in deep self-mistrust let us approach these " dim discovered tracks of mind," baffling profoundest intellects heretofore, perhaps now to be laid clear ; leading, let us hope, to precious stores, that are not to be blunderingly rifled, but by discerning handicraft to be drawn and sifted as the ruby, emerald, and the diamond mines.

" Seek and ye shall find, knock, and it shall be opened unto you."

Noscere sese, et quæ sibi sit cælestis origo,
    Hæc via, quæ superas ducit adire domos.

" What tho' in solemn silence all,
Move round our dark terrestrial ball,
What tho' no outward voice nor sound
Amid their radiant orbs be found,
In *Reason's ear* they all rejoice,
And utter *still* their glorious voice ;
For ever singing, as they shine,
The *Hand* that moves *Us* is *Divine*."

But all are now statistical, archæological, when the great problem, the mind of man had yet to be unsolved, and why ? the case was in-

tricate, and cobwebs coarse, and finest webs of
sophistry have been woven around it ; truth
plain and palpable has stalked away from us, and
before us ; but a new power is developing itself,
growing in its strength ; let us with due knowledge seek its aid, and in these latter days let us
ask for fresh and bold abettors in the cause.

> " Parvas ecce MANUS *vagabundis* offero *turmis,*
> Unius quia vana est, et sine viribus ira ;
> Difficile ac durum est unum compescere multos.
> Hei mihi ! quam parvi levis est vindicta lacerti !
> Non ego, quod veniam novus ignotusque sacerdos
> Gratus ero fortasse minus.
>
> Facta cano, sed erunt qui me finxisse loquentur
> Credite, qui terrena volunt, cælestia nolunt,
> Qui ad terram accedit, cælum fugit, æthera amare
> Nemo potest, nisi sit terreno exutus amore."

The present address, however, might not
have been called forth at the present moment,
but for the announcement of a phenomenon in
the western horizon ; here fettered as we are by
our old and unaspiring institutions, it is deemed
but rashly starting on the forlorn hope to pass
the lines, or quit for simple truth's unprofitable
field, the well accoutred camp ; but now to " go
a head" seems to be the acknowledged watch-
word of young America ; and there in such a

spirit, (reckless though we call it) ere long perchance a splendour, a broad meteor, is destined
to arise.

* Poe   The announcement lately made by Mr. Poe (Poe
whose examination of his sleep waker on a *previous*
occasion, is certainly, supposing it genuine, the
most remarkable and deeply interesting of any yet
recorded) of a dying man magnetised by him in
articulo mortis, and though inevitable death did
certainly supervene, yet there in his chamber and
in testimony of a crowd of witnesses, for seven
months consecutively lay the undemagnetised
corpse, and when questioned by the magnetiser
Poe, in a sepulchral voice gave utterance that he
was dead, dead, and should not be disturbed; and
then, when at the intervention of others, Poe made
the demagnetising passes, the outward body,
the whole perfect form instantly dissolved into
one shapeless mass of intolerable corruption.
This is well and publicly attested, yet few even
of the faithful will believe, though one spoke
from the dead.   But be it true or false to this
generation, " Ye shall see greater things than
these."

The immediate object having chiefly been to
adduce several texts and passages from sacred
scripture more particularly bearing on the evidently very ancient practice of Magnetism, I

shall forbear to enlarge on the subject in the
present state of the science and lagging reception
of it, and shall not now proceed, although the
task were easy to cite the allusions almost infinite in every type and metaphor, (without the
key shut up in darkness) scattered throughout
and long admired, (though little light was on
them) the deep adored inestimable gems of holy
writ, not without cause so valued ; the inner eye
had caught some sparklings of their lustre, and
outward sense devotionally raised, delighted and
refined, and wrapt by verbal sound, and drawing from the responsive glow within, have
sometime kindled into light and tasted joy, surpassing visual rays, far as etherial hallowing
intellectual flame outshines the elemental fire.

" Sicut flamma mari differt, et sydera terrâ."

Nor let us vainly think we have attained
before, or now, to sources unexplored by pious
seers in days more bright than ours ; for verily
in chrystal truth to see, there is one only medium
through all worlds, whereat when proud philosophy has duly learned to bow, she may in one
short hour attain to more than all this long
experimenting age has taught her. Now may
we read with understanding how Solomon would

teach us Wisdom, nor should we all despair ; the gate more open than before admits us ;

> " Salubrious Pæon blossoms into light,
> Health far diffusing, and th' extended world
> With streams of harmony innoxious fills."

And the star leads on ; we needed but this spark to catch the dry parched waste of life : 'tis smothering yet, but be ye well prepared to watch and bear the blaze. An all wise Providence is surely round, directing that it purely burn, and will in mercy stay the strong ordeal, that it but come to save, not to destroy.

Finally let me once more with a warning voice recur, as expressed in sacred allegory, to the holy ground we tread on. And should it yet be asked by any what is the meaning of that phrase ? Let me say, it is what only and alone the trance presents, the sabbath of the senses ; deep inner retirement from the every day routine of worldly thoughts and occupations, for central self-communion ; to feel, to see and know the yet unstirred, unapproached, unappreciated, unbelieved, unrevered *Divinity* within us ; to waken up the buried Conscience like a Guardian Spirit, starting in beautiful relief from out the flat, dull, unprofitable, monotonous picture com-

mon life presents ; to pass into a freer state of
being imagined only by the high aspiring minds
glancing at the shadow, but well described and
dwelt upon by those who verily and in truth
have rested on this ground. Believe it all the
great philosophic masters from Thales to Aris-
totle, from Orpheus down to Virgil, including
his yet bright more modern name, and Homer
his more bright original, aye may I say, allowing no exceptions, every truly inspired originating
mind from Adam to this hour, all have known
this *terram incognitam* to the many, but *firmissi-
mam* to the happier few? Those perchance at
times and at their leisure, only having drawn
pleasure from the bare reflection of what these
had been in close communion with as part and
parcel of their being.

As this magnetic key has in all humility
been thus applied to the two master wards
of the Old Testament, and should it, as we
have thought in this instance, seem to open
the way, as surely may we hope reverently and
not vainly to apply it to the golden treasures of
the New.

" Know ye not that ye are the Temple of
God ?"

But let us hesitate in awe and diffidence, and ask, is the time yet rife for such a bursting, dazzling, deep, devotional blaze of revealment?

Are we in this latter time prepared? We ask and pause for a reply; and in the busy darkness all around, the faithful monitor within, but echoes the response,

Pause for a reply.

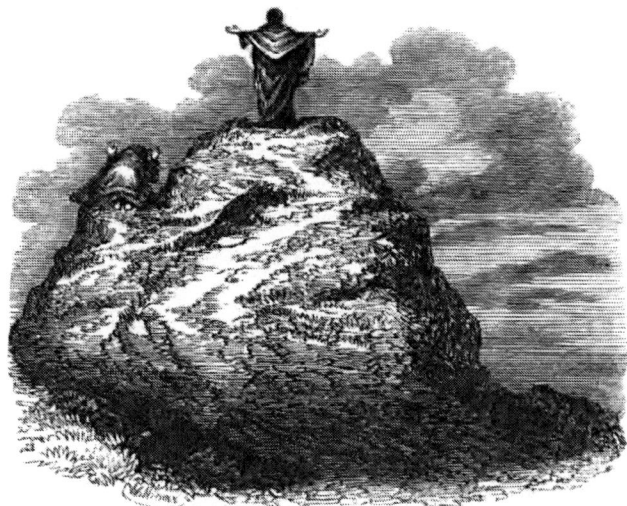

Startled, awake ye dreamers ! look to the beacon, and ask ye,
  Ask, is it even so ? come to the mount and behold !
Trembling come and attend the behest of the Prophet on
      Carmel.
  See ye the rising cloud ? See ye the hand in the cloud ?
See ye the storm in the hand, and the blessing of rain for the
      thirsty ?
  Haste for a swooping flood cometh, ye may not abide.
But, ere yet ye descend, look well to the omen, it carries
  (Even the hand in the cloud) light, may ye catch it, divine.
See if prosperity pour through every jet in the city,
  If in the growing fields all, but contentment, abound.
Yea, it is even so ; look well to the signs, and be sure the
  Greatness is ripening, all ready to reap, or to burn.
Think ye the harvest ripe ? be sure ye look to the harvest,
  Ripe for the sickle ; and self, e'en as the moon at the full

Standeth learning at bay ? and science aghast at her wonders ?
    Have we clomb to the high zenith of arts and of arms ?
Are the projectiles ready ? the last new patent projectiles,
    Once more havoc ! and once more to the vulture ye cry !
Will ye be brave once more, and away from the ball to the
        battle ?
    Hear ye the warder's blast, soundeth the trumpet afar ?
Have we the brimful measure ? the cornucopia flowing !
    Reeking foul doth the world steam with iniquity ? doth
Every vice stand high on every precipice ? topling
    Goats ! are the sheep fast bound bleating and bleeding for
        Baal ?
When it is climax all, one Mammon worship ; we travel
    Fast to the goal, friends, fast ! faster, for there shall be
        signs ;
Then it is written, behold ! in mercy the time shall be shorten'd,
    There shall be signs, for the Lord cometh, and there shall
        be signs.
O ! then open, ye Gates, for the king shall enter in glory !
    Open, ye golden Doors, lift up your Heads, O ye Gates !
Every knee bow down, <u>shut every sense,</u> in his holy
    Temple the Lord of Hosts cometh, for thus saith the Lord.

APPENDIX.

" Quis monstrum ? Ille pius Chiron," &c.

Who then is this ? He the good Chiron, *the* Hand-worker, above all the cloud-descended race, and Tutor of the great Achilles.

" Felices, animæ," &c.

Fortunate those souls whose care it first has been to gain knowledge of these things, so as to climb up to the celestial abodes. Doubtless they also have been able to lift the mind up from vice and frivolity high over human concerns.

" Sume fidem et pharetram," &c.

> Take then the Lyre, and bend the Bow,
>   Apollo manifested be.
> Lo ! golden horns now grace thy brow,
>   Thou Bacchanalian deity !

" Tunc ire ad mundum archetypum," &c.

Then have we free access to the Archetypal World ; to go often, and to return, and to behold the Father of All.

" O quam te dicam bonam," &c.

Oh ! how good shall I pronounce thee to have been formerly, since such are thy remains !

" Illis viva acies hec pupula," &c.

> Theirs is the living light, the holy fire,
>   (No little sensual pupil of the eye,)
> Transporting through all space the free desire,
>   And boundless blending with Infinity.

" Sed fortasse aliquis quærit."

But some one would ask, perhaps, what is Wisdom? Assuredly it is no other than Causal knowledge, by which the pure mind, (weighed down by no human burden, and free from earthly affections), climbs the heights of Heaven, and in Olympus mingles with the Gods, despising all things mortal; like to the Fire, ever aspiring still on High. " 'Tis Athenæa! child of Zeus supreme. The ægis-holder, on her father's floor, clothed in her peplus various, laboured with her hands, the tunic of the cloud-collecting Zeus, fitted for *tearful* war. Around her shoulder cast is that fringed Ægis which all about is compassed with fear; in it is Strife, in it is Strength, and in it chill Pursuit; in it the Gorgon head, the portent dire and terrific, the great Prodigy. See on her head the four coned casque of gold, fitting the footmen of a hundred towns; the flaming car she mounts, and grasps the spear, great, heavy, solid, wherewith, when she is wroth, the strong sired maiden whole ranks of heroes vanquisheth."

" Non bene tractantur musæ," &c.

The Muses incline not to public communion, nor are they drawn in the broad sun-light; they shun the motley throng; the laughing gaze and empty wits of men. The crowd, the streets, the open air passed by, then will the Muses come and yield a copious harvest.

" Palmaque nobilis," &c.

And the noble *Palm* lifts up the Lords of Earth to the Gods on High!

" Hæc via scintillans sublustri," &c.

This sparkling way disclosed through glimmering night most brilliant with innumerable stars in the clear heaven, Elysian, and all sapphirine ; this leads us to the Manes' shades, and happy fields, and to the secret throne. Here in the vast concave, with lighted torches, do the Good proclaim Eternal Glory night and day. Neither do I fear (allowing but the due poetic licence), to call this the High Olympus and the Court of Jove.

" Caligo hæc ingens," &c.

This thick darkness, forbidding you to know the truth, at once remove ; your eyes will then behold better things ; and those things which you now may esteem great goods, perhaps you may then deny to be good at all, and those you now believe the greatest evils, perchance you will esteem quite otherwise. The cloud once cast away from off your heart, there springs up that clear light of mind, which sees within whatever lay concealed ; whoever uses this judges of all things rightly, and he will witness wonders.

" Omnia jam fiunt fieri," &c.

All things are now being done, that still are denied to be possible, and what is there to which we may not lend our faith ?

" Quare non mirum est," &c.

No wonder if the world give little credence to these words ; verily their minds are most obtuse. Biped moles, continually buried deep in earth, never with uplifted sight beholding heaven.

" Corpus sed carceris instar," &c.

But the body is the prison of the mind, which it enfolds with strength of limb, stifling its etherial keen light, as the earthen vessel dims the flame whose fire burns within.

" Natus humo despectat humum," &c.

The earth-born nature still looks down to earth, seeking terrestrial things with its whole heart, and knows not what it is to look for wealth in heaven, like the poor bramble which, having spread far forth its branches on high, bends down, and with its topmost shoot again upon the ground, once more is rooted.

" Ergo felices vivunt nectarque," &c.

There do the blessed live, and drinking nectar, feed on green ambrosia, which every where and in abundance, springs in the celestial fields ; but such things to the world are all unknown, nor will the common herd believe them. And what of that ? Wherefore throw pearls to swine ? Believe them, O ! ye Wise ? Do you of higher mind *believe !* But not to all is it allowed to *know* such mysteries divine. These things are perceived by few, approved by the Creator, pouring on them his own Light proper for such contemplations. Therefore let us first begin our work by being cleansed, and purified, and clarified to the nail ; throwing off this dross, and casting the foul cloak away, that we may shine forth all beautiful in snowy virgin virtue.

" Noscere sese et quæ sibi sit," &c.

To know ourselves, and what celestial origin we come of, is the way that leads us to the seats above.

" Parvas ecce manus vagabundis," &c.

Behold I offer these little Hands, (*" vagabundis turmis"* is too truly *British* to require or admit of translation), for the wrath of one is of no force. 'Tis hard and difficult for one to hold in check the many; How small is the resistance of the light lizard against the throng! Perchance I may not be the less welcome coming as a fresh and unknown servitor in truth's good cause.

" *Facta cano, sed erunt qui me,*" &c.

I speak of facts, but there are those who will think I tell them fables. Believe me, they whose cares are earthly, turn from things celestial. He who is attracted to earth is far from heaven; no one can be drawn up with love divine unless he have thrown off worldly affections.

" *Sicut flamma mari differt,*" &c.

Far as is pain from pleasure, grief from mirth,
As fire from water, or as heaven from earth.

END.

LONDON:
Printed by Schulze and Co., 13, Poland Street.

SUPPLÉMENT AU CATALOGUE

DE LA

LIBRAIRIE SCIENTIFIQUE,

ANGLAISE, FRANÇAISE, ET ALLEMANDE,

DE

H. BAILLIÈRE,

FOREIGN BOOKSELLER TO THE ROYAL COLLEGE OF SURGEONS, AND THE ROYAL MEDICAL AND CHIRURGICAL SOCIETY OF LONDON,

219 REGENT STREET, LONDON.

H. B. continues to receive a weekly parcel from France, containing the newest Works on Science and General Literature, which he supplies at One Shilling per Franc on the advertised Price at Paris. He begs to acquaint his friends, and the patrons of German Scientific Works, that he is able to furnish German Works and Periodicals every Month at the rate of Four Shillings the Rix-Dollar.

ABICH. Ueber die Natur und den Gusammenhang der Vulkanischen Bildungen. 4to. mit 3 cartes, 2 planches. Braunschweig, 1841. 18s.

—— Vues Illustratives de quelques Phénomènes Géologiques prises sur le Vésuve et l'Etna, pendant les années 1833 et 1834. Folio. Paris, 20s.

ABLES. Erläuterungen zur Allgemeinen Pathologie. 8vo. Wien, 1844. 9s.

ACHARIUS. Methodus quo omnes detectos Lichenes secundum Organa Carpomorpha ad Genera, Species, et Varietates redigere atque observationibus illustrare. With 8 coloured plates. 8vo. Stockholmiæ, 1803. 15s.

ACKERMAN. Considérations Anatomico - Physiologiques et Historiques sur le Coïpo du Chili. 4to. avec 3 planches. Paris, 1844. 3s.

AGARDH (C. A.) Ueber die Eintheilung der Pflanzen nach den Katyledonen. With a plate. 4to. 2s. 6d.

—— Ueber die Anatomie und den Kreislauf der Charen. With a coloured plate. 4to. 2s.

—— Icones Algarum Europæarum. 8vo. with 40 coloured plates. Leipsic, 1828. 1l. 8s.

—— Synopsis Generis Lupini. 8vo. with a plate. 2s. 6d.

—— Systema Algarum. 12mo. Lundæ, 1824. 12s.

—— Species Algarum. 2 vols. 8vo. Gryphiæ, 1821–28. 1l. 7s.

AGASSIZ. Monographie des Poissons Fossiles du vieux Grès Rouge, ou Système Dévonien (old red sandstone) des Iles Britanniques et de Russie. Supplemens aux Poissons Fossiles. Deux livraisons fol. de 26 planches, et texte. 4to. Neufchâtel, 1844. 3l.

—— Recherches sur les Poissons Fossiles, comprenant la description de 500 espèces qui n'existent plus, l'exposition des lois de la succession et du développement organique des poissons, nouvelle classification de ces animaux, exprimant leur rapport, avec la série des formations ; enfin des considérations géologiques générales, tirées de l'étude de ces fossiles. Neufchâtel, 1833–43, 5 vol. in-4, et atlas de 250 pl. in folio, publiés en 18 livraisons. Prix de chaque livraison, 1l. 10s. Ouvrage complet.

Les livraisons 13 à 18, to complete sets, can be had separately.

ALLIONIUS. Flora Pedemontana, sive enumeratio methodica stirpium indigenarum Pedemontii. 2 vols. folio, plates. 1775. 1l. 10s.

AMMANO. Stirpium Rariorum in Imperio Rutheno sponte provenientium Icones et Descriptiones. 35 plates. 4to. Petropoli, 1789. 6s. 6d.

AMMON. Die Angeborenen chirurgischen Krankheiten des Menschen. Avec un atlas de 34 planches, folio and text. Berlin, 1842. 3l.

—— Klinische Darstellungen der Krankheiten des menschlichen Auges. Fol. mit 55 ill. Kupfern. Berlin, 1838–41. 7l. 12s.

ANALEKTEN über Kinderkrankheiten oder sammlung Auserwahlter Abhandlungen über die Krankheiten des Kindlichen alters. 4 vols. 8vo. Stuttgart, 1834. 1l.

ANATOMY. The Edinburgh Dissector. System of Practical Anatomy, for the use of Students in the Dissecting-Room. By a Fellow of the College of Surgeons in Edinburgh. 12mo. London, 1837. 9s.

ANDRAL. Cours de Pathologie interne, professé à la Faculté de Médecine de Paris. 8vo. 10s. 6d.

—— Precis d'Anatomie Pathologique. 3 vols. 8vo. Paris, 1829. 18s.

ANDRY. Manuel Pratique de Percussion et d'Auscultation. 12mo. Paris, 1844. 3s. 6d.

ANNALES d'Oculistique et de Gynecologie, publiés par F. Cunier. Vol. I. in-4. Bruxelles, 1838. 18s. Vols. II.–XII. in-8. Bruxelles, 1833-1844. 5l.

—— d'Hygiène publique et de Médecine Légale, par MM. Adelon, Andral, d'Arcet, Barruel, Chevallier, Devergie, Esquirol, Gaultier de Claubry, Guerard, Keraudren, Leuret, Marc, Ollivier (d'Angers), Orfila, Parent-Duchatelet, Trebuchet, Villerme. Les Annales d'Hygiène publique et de Médecine Légale paraissent depuis 1829 régulièrement tous les trois mois par cahiers in-8, 250 pages, avec des planches. Le prix de l'abonnement, par an, est de 1l. 4s.

La collection complète 1829 à 1844, dont il ne reste que peu d'exemplaires. 32 vol. in-8, fig. Prix 14l. 14s.

Tables Alphabétiques par ordre des matières et par noms d'auteurs des Tomes I. à XX. pour 1829 à 1838, in-8. 2s. 6d.

CAVANILLES (A. J.) Observaciones sobre el historia natural geografía, agricultura, poblacion y frutos der Reyno de Valencia. 4to. 2 vol. in 1. With maps and views. Madrid, 1795. 3*l.*

CAZENAVE (A.) Traité des Syphilides, ou maladies vénériennes de la peau. In-8, et atlas de 12 planches in-folio, gravées et coloriées. Paris, 1843. 1*l.* 14*s.*

—— Abrégé Pratique des Maladies de la Peau d'après les Documens pensés dans les leçons cliniques de M. le Docteur BIETT. 1 vol. 8vo. Paris, 1838. 11*s.*

CHAPMAN. A Brief Description of the Characters of Minerals; forming a familiar Introduction to the Science of Mineralogy. 1 vol. 12mo. With 3 plates. London, 1844. 4*s.*

—— Practical Mineralogy; or, a Compendium of the Distinguishing Characters of Minerals. By which the name of any species or variety in the mineral kingdom may be speedily ascertained. Illustrated with 13 engravings, shewing 270 specimens. 8vo. London, 1843. 7*s.*

CHARPENTIER. Libellulinæ Europæ descriptæ, et depictæ cum tabulis 48 coloratis. 4to. Leipsig, 1840. 3*l.* 4*s.*

CHERFBERR. Rapport à M. le ministre de l'intérieur sur différens hôpitaux, hospices, établissemens et sociétés de bienfaisance de l'Italie. In-4. Paris, 1840. 15*s.*

CHEVREUL. A fine Portrait of. Folio. 5*s.*

CHIRURGISCHE Hand-Bibliothek. Eine Auserlesene Sammlung der besten neueren Chirurgischen Schriften des Auslandes. 14 bde. 8vo. kupf. Wiemar, 1824-37. 3*l.*

CHOULANT (L.) Vorlesung über die Kranioskopie oder Schädellehre. 8vo. Dresden, 1844. 2*s.* 6*d.*

CLOQUET (J.) Manuel complet d'anatomie descriptive du Corps Humain. 3 vol. in-4, avec 340 planches. Paris, 1835. Fig. noires, 8*l.*; fig. col. 15*l.*

COATES (M.) Practical Observations on the Nature and Treatment of the Talipes, or Club-Foot; particularly of the Talipes Verus. With 2 plates. 8vo. London, 1840. 2*s.* 6*d.*

COMMELIN. Horti Medici Rariorum Plantarum descriptio et icones. 2 vols. fol. planches. Amstelodami, 1697. 1*l.*

—— Icones Plantarum, quaquaversum præsertim ex Indiis, Collectarum, with 84 plates. 4to. Lugd. Batav. 1715. 6*s.*

COMOLLIO (J.) Plantarum in Lariensi Provincia Lectarum. Enumeratio quam ipse in Botaniphilorum usu atque commodo eschebet uti Prodromum Floræ comensis. 8vo. New edition. 1824. 8*s.*

COOPER (SIR ASTLEY). Œuvres chirurgicales complètes, traduites de l'Anglais, avec des notes par CHASSAIGNAC et RICHELOT. 8vo. Paris, 1837. 14*s.*

COQUEBERT. Illustratio iconographia insectorum quæ in musæis Parisinis observavit et in lucem edidit J. CH. FABRICIUS, præmisais ejusdem descriptionibus accedent species plurimæ, vel minus aut nondum cognitæ. Parisiis, an viii. in-4, de 142 pages de texte, et 30 pl. gravées et coloriées avec soin et réprésentant plus de 300 espèces. 1 vol. in-4, cart. 3*l.*

COURTENAY (F. B.) On the Pathology and Cure of Stricture in the Urethra; Illustrating, by a selection from numerous interesting facts and cases, the Origin, Progress, and History of this Disease, in all its Phases, and embracing every variety of Morbid Contraction to which the Urethra is liable, together with an account of the mode of treatment successfully adopted in each case: thus forming a complete Practical Manual and Guide to the Appropriate Treatment and Cure of every species of Urethral Stricture. The whole followed by some Observations on the Chronic Enlargement of the Prostate Gland in Old Men, and its Treatment. Third edition. 8vo. London, 1845. 7*s.* 6*d.*

—— Practical Observations on the Chronic Enlargement of the Prostate Gland in Old People, with Mode of Treatment. Containing numerous cases and plates. 8vo, in boards. London, 1839. 7*s.* 6*d.*

CRAMER (P.) Papillons exotiques des trois parties du monde, l'Asie, l'Afrique, et l'Amérique. 4 vol. in-4, et un supplément par STOLL, avec 400 pl. coloriées, reliés. Amsterdam, 1779. 20*l.*

CRANTZ (J. N.) Stirpium Austriacarum. 4to. fig. Vienne, 1769. 12*s.*

CRUVEILHIER. Anatomie du système nerveux de l'homme. Partie I. Folio, avec 2 planches. Paris, 1838. 6*s.*

—— Anatomie pathologique du corps humain, ou descriptions avec figures lithographiées et coloriées des diverses altérations morbides dont le corps humain est susceptible. Ouvrage complet, publié en 41 liv. chacune contenant 6 feuilles de texte grand in-fol. raisin vélin, avec 5 pl. color. et 6 pl. lorsqu'il n'y a que 4 pl. color. Paris, 1830-1842. 22*l.* 11*s.*

Subscribers are requested to complete their set, as in a few months the Publisher will not guarantee to be able to do so.

—— Anatomie descriptive. Seconde édit. 4 vol. in-8. Paris, 1843. 1*l.* 8*s.*

—— Atlas of the Descriptive Anatomy of the Human Body, with Explanation by C. BONAMY. Vol. I. containing 82 4to. plates of Osteology, Syndemology, and Myology. Plain, 3*l.*; coloured, 5*l.* London, 1844.

—— Atlas Illustrative of the Anatomy of the Human Body. Drawn from Nature by M. E. BEAU, with Description by M. G. BONAMY, M.D. This *Atlas* will consist altogether of 200 plates, small 4to. and is published in Numbers, each containing 4 plates, with descriptions, to be continued monthly until the completion. 2*s.* 6*d.* plain; coloured, 5*s.* (Parts I. to XXII. are out.)

Extract from a letter of Professor CRUVEILHIER to H. BAILLIÈRE, dated Paris, June 10, 1841:—

"*Je déclare que les Planches sont extrêmement remarquables par leur exactitude, et par les soins avec lesquelles elles sont exécutées. Je me propose d'y renvoyer toujours dans* (LA 2e ÉDITION DE) MON ANATOMIE DESCRIPTIVE!
(Signed) "J. CRUVEILHIER."

CURIE (P. F.) Annals of the London Homœopathic Dispensary. 1 vol. 8vo. 20 Nos. 1841-42. 15*s.*

—— Practice of Homœopathy. 1 vol. 8vo. London, 1838. 6*s.*

—— Principles of Homœopathy. 1 vol. 8vo. London, 1837. 5*s.*

—— Domestic Homœopathy. Third edit. 12mo. London, 1844. 5*s.*

See JAHR.

CURTIS AND LILLIE. An Epitome of Homœopathic Practice; compiled chiefly from JAHR, RUCKERT, BEAUVAIS, BÖNNINGHAUSEN. 12mo. New York, 1843. 5*s.*

CUVIER. A fine Portrait of. 3*s.* 6*d.*

—— Iconographie du règne animal de G. CUVIER, ou réprésentation d'après nature de l'une des espèces le plus rémarquables, et souvent non encore figurée de chaque genre d'animaux, ouvrage pouvant servir d'atlas à tous les traités de zoologie, par F. E. GUÉRIN, membre de diverses sociétés savantes nationales et étrangères. Paris, 1830-44. 7 vol. grand in-8. Ce bel ouvrage est complet. Il a été publié en 50 livraisons, chacune de 10 planches gravées. 2 vol. 8vo. de texte. Prix de chaque livraison, in-8, figures noires, 6*s.*

—— Le même, in-8, fig. col. 15*s.*
—— Le même, in-4, fig. col. 1*l.*

L'ouvrage complet est composé de 450 planches, avec un texte explicatif pour chacune des divisions qui se vendent séparément in-8, savoir:

	pl.	fig. n.	fig. col.		
1°. Mammifères, avec le portrait de G. CUVIER	53	1	12	4	0
2°. Oiseaux	70	2	2	5	3
3°. Reptiles	30	0	18	2	3
4°. Poissons	70	2	2	5	3
5°. Mollusques et zoophytes	63	1	18	4	15
6°. Annélides, crustacés, et arachnides	53	1	12	4	0
7°. Insectes, avec le portrait de LATREILLE	111	3	6	8	5

CUVIER. Iconographie du Règne Animal, 46e à 50e liv. (Texte par GUÉRIN). 2 vols. 8vo. Paris, 1844. 30s.
—— Leçons d'Anatomie comparée, publiées par DUMÉRIL, LAURILLARD, et DUVERNOY. Seconde édition. 10 vol. in-8. Paris, 1835-43. Les Tomes I. II. IV. (Parties I. II.) V. VI. VII. sont en vente. Prix de chaque, 7s.
—— Tableau élémentaire d'histoire naturelle des animaux. In-8. Rare. Paris, an vii. 16s.
D'ALTON. Die Skelete der Straussartigen Vögel abgebildet und beschrieben, ufol. with 7 plates. Bonn, 1827. 1l. 10s.
DAMBERGER, Sechzig Genealogische auch Chronologische, u. Statische, Tabellen zu Fürstentafel und Fürstenbuch, der europäischen Staatengeschichte. Folio. Regensburg, 1831. 10s.
DAVEY (J. G.) Medico-Legal Reflections on the Trial of DANIEL M'NAUGHTEN, for the Murder of Mr. DRUMMOND; with Remarks on the different Forms of Insanity and the Irresponsibility of the Insane. 8vo. London, 1843. 1s. 6d.
DE CANDOLLE. Prodromus Systemati Naturalis Regni Vegetabilis. 8 vols. 8vo. Paris, 1824-44. 5l. 17s.
—— Index generalis et specialis ad Prodromum Systematis Naturalis Regni Vegetabilis. Edidit H. W. BUEK, M.D. 8vo. Berlin, 1842. 1l.
—— Collection de Mémoires pour servir à l'histoire du règne végétal. 8 mémoires, in-4, avec 80 planches. 3l.
DEGEER. Abhandlungen zur Geschichte der Insecten, übersetzt von GOEZE. 7 bde. 4to. kupf. 4l. 10s.
DEJEAN. Spécies Général des Coléoptères. 6 vol. in-8. Paris, 1825-38. 6l.
DEMANGEON. Physiologie Intellectuelle, ou l'Esprit de l'Homme. Troisième Edition, enrichi de plusieurs Observations nouvelles. 1 vol. in-8. Paris, 1843. 8s.
DESCRIPTION des principaux parcs et jardins de l'Europe, avec des remarques sur le jardinage et les plantations, ouvrage enrichi d'estampes coloriées. 3 vols. fol. 6l. 6s.
DESFONTAINES. Flora Atlantica, sive Historia Plantarum quæ in Atlante, agro Tunetano, et Algeriensi, &c. 2 vol. in-4, avec 263 planches, gravées d'après les dessins de REDOUTÉ. Parisiis, 1798. 3l. 10s.
DESIRABODE. Nouveaux Eléments complets de la Science et de l'Art du Dentiste. 2 vol. in-8. Paris, 1843. 14s.
DESOR. Excursions et séjours dans les glaciers et les hautes régions des Alpes de M. AGASSIZ et de ses compagnons de voyage. In-12, 5 plates. Neuchâtel, 1844. 9s. 6d.
DEVAL (CHARLES). Chirurgie Oculaire, ou Traité des Opérations Chirurgicales sur l'Œil. 1 vol. in-8. Paris, 1844. 8s.
DEVERGIE. Clinique de la Maladie Syphilitique. 2 vol. in-4, atlas de 150 planches coloriées. Paris, 1823. 7l. 7s.
—— (ALPH.) Médecine légale, théorique et pratique, avec le Texte et l'Interpretation des lois relatives à la Médecine légale, revus et annotés par J. B. DEHAUSSY, conseiller à la Cour de Cassation. Deuxième édition, augmentée. 3 vol. in-8. Paris, 1840. 1l. 1s.
DIERBACH. Die neuesten Eutdeckungen, in der Materia Medica. 1 vol. 8vo. Leipzig, 1840. 12s.
DICTIONNAIRE Raisonné, étymologique, synonymique et polyglotte, des termes usités dans les Sciences Naturelles, comprenant l'anatomie, l'histoire naturelle et la physiologie générales, l'astronomie, la botanique, la chimie, la géographie physique, la géologie, la minéralogie, la physique, la zoologie, &c.; par A. J. L. JOURDAN. 2 forts vol. in-8, petite-texte à 2 colonnes. Paris, 1834. 18s.
—— universal de Matière médicale et de Thérapeutique générale, contenant l'indication, la description et l'emploi de tous les Médicamens connus dans les diverses parties du Globe, &c. par MM. MÉRAT et DELENS, membres de l'Académie royale de médecine. Ouvrage complet. 6 forts vol. in-8. Paris, 1829-34. 2l. 12s.

DICTIONNAIRE des sciences médicales, par MM. ALARD, ALIBERT, BOYER, CHAUSSIER, CUVIER, GARDIEN, HALLE, MARJOLIN, MÉRAT, NYSTEN, PINEL, ROUX, ROYER-COLLARD, VIREY. 60 vol. in-8, half-bound. Paris, 1812-22. 18l. 18s.
—— de l'industrie manufacturière, commerciale, et agricole, ouvrage accompagné de 1200 figures intercalées dans le texte, par MM. BAUDRIMONT, BLANQUI, COLLADIN, CORIOLIS, D'ARCET, P. DESORMEAUX, DESPRETS, H. GAULTIER DE CLAUBRY, GOURLIER, TH. OLIVIER, PARENT-DUCHATELET, SAINTE-PREUVE, SOULANGE-BODIN, TREBOUCHET, &c. Ouvrage complet. 10 vol. in-8, de 700 pp. chacun. Paris, 1834-41. Prix de chaque, 8s.
—— De Médecine et de Chirurgie pratiques, par MM. ANDRAL, BEGIN, BLANDIN, BOUILLAUD, BOUVIER, CRUVEILHIER, CULLERIER, DESLANDES, DEVERGIE, DUGÈS, DUPUYTREN, FOVILLE, GUIBOURT, JOLLY, LALLEMAND, LONDE, MAGENDIE, MARTIN-SOLON, RATIER, RAYER, ROCHE, ET SANSON. Ouvrage complet. 15 forts vol. in-8. Paris, 1829-36. Le prix de chaque volume est de 7s.
DIEFFENBACH. Die Operative Chirurgie. 2 parts. 8vo. Leipzig, 1844. 8s.
DIOSCORIDIS Anazarbei, de materia medica libri quinque, ad fidem manuscriptorum et cum commentariis illustravit C. SPRENGEL, Grece et Latine. 2 vols. 8vo. Lipsiæ, 1829. 1l. 10s.
DIETRICH (D.) Das Wichtigste aus dem Pflanzenreiche für Landwirthe, Fabrikanten, Forst-und Schulmänner, so wie für Liebhaber der Pflanzenkunde überhaupt. 22 parts, small folio, each containing 4 col. plates. Jena, 1831-38. 2l.
—— Deutschlands Kryptogamische Gewächse. Parts I. and II. 8vo. with 26 col. pls. each. Jena, 1843. 1l.
—— Synopsis Plantarum. 3 vols. 8vo. Vinariæ, 1839. 3l. 16s.
—— (A.) Flora Marchica oder Beschreibung der in der Mark Brandenburg wildwachsenden Pflanzen. 12mo. Berlin, 1841. 12s.
DIETERICHS (J. F. C.) Berträge zur Veterinar-Chirurgie und Akiurgie. 8vo. with plates. Berlin, 1844. 4s.
DISSERTATION sur le cacao et le café et le thé, sur leur culture et sur les différentes préparations. Fol. avec 7 planches coloriées. 8s.
DONNE (A.) Cours de Microscopie complémentaire des études médicales, anatomie, microscopique, et physiologie des fluides de l'économie. In-8. Paris, 1844. 7s. 6d.
D'ORBIGNY. Voyage dans l'Amérique Méridionale, partie Paléontologie. In-4, avec 22 planches. Paris, 1843. 2l. 5s.
—— Voyage dans l'Amérique Méridionale, partie Géologie. In-4, avec 11 planches coloriées. Paris, 1843. 3l. 15s.
—— L'Homme Américain (de l'Amérique Méridionale), considéré sous les rapports physiologiques et moraux. 2 vol. in-8, avec un atlas de 15 planches in-4. Paris, 1839. 18s.
DUBRUNFAUT. Traité complet de l'art de la distillation. 2 vol. in-8. Paris, 1824. 18s. Very scarce.
—— Art de fabriquer de sucre de Betteraves. In-8, 1825. 9s.
DUCPETIAUX de la Mortalité à Bruxelles, comparée à celle des autres grandes villes. In-8, with a map. Bruxelles, 1844. 4s.
—— de la condition physique et moral des jeunes ouvriers et des moyens de l'améliorer. 2 vol. in-8. Bruxelles. 16s.
DUFRENOY (A.) Traité de minéralogie. 2 vols. with plates. In-8. Paris, 1844. 18s.
DUGES. Traité de physiologie comparée de l'homme et des animaux. 3 vol. in-8. avec planches lithographiées. Montpelier, 1838. 24s.
DUMAS, a fine portrait of. Folio. 5s.
—— Traité de Chimie appliquée aux arts. Vol. VII. in-8. Paris, 1844. 12s. 6d.
DUMAS AND BOUSSINGAULT. The Chemical and Physiological Balance of Organic Nature; an Essay. 12mo. London, 1844. 4s.
See BOUSSINGAULT.

DUMORTIER (C.) Essai carpographique présentant une nouvelle classification des fruits. 4to. with 4 plates. Bruxelles, 1835. 6s.

DUNAL. Considerations sur la Nature et les rapports de quelques uns des Organes de la fleur. In-4, avec 3 planches. Paris, 1829. 8s.

—— Monographie de la famille des annonacées. 4to. 25 plates. Paris, 1817. 1l. 5s.

DUNSFORD (H.) The Practical Advantages of Homœopathy, illustrated by numerous Cases. Dedicated by permission to Her Majesty Queen Adelaide. 1 vol. 8vo. boards. 1841. 8s.

—— The Pathogenetic Effects of some of the principal Homœopathic Remedies. 8vo. London, 1838. 9s.

DUPASQUIER. Traité élémentaire de chimie industrielle. 1 vol. in-8. Paris, 1844. 9s.

DUSING (Dr. August). Krystallinsensystem des Menschlichen Auges. In-8. Berlin, 1844. 5s.

DUTROCHET. Mémoires pour servir à l'histoire anatomique et physiologique des Végétaux et des Animaux. Avec cette épigraphe : "Je considère comme non avenu tout ce que j'ai publié précédemment sur ces matières, et qui ne se trouve point reproduit dans cette collection." Paris, 1837. 2 vol. in-8, accompagnés d'un atlas de 30 planches gravées. Paris, 1837. 1l. 4s.

EBERS (J. J. H.) Die Ehe und die Ehegesetze vom naturwissenschaftlichen Standpuncte beleuchtet. 8vo. Erlangen, 1844. 2s. 6d.

EHRENBERG. Zusatze zur Erkenntniss Grosser Organisation im Kleinen Raume. Folio, with 1 coloured plate. Berlin, 1836. 6s.

—— Zur Erkenntniss der Organisation in der Richtung des Kleinsten Raumes. 4to. with 4 plates. Berlin, 1842. 1l.

—— Organisation in der Richtung des Kleinsten Raumes. 4to. with 11 coloured plates. Berlin, 1834. 1l. 10s.

—— (C. G.) Die Infusionsthierchen als vollkommene Organismen. 1 vol. folio, with 64 col. plates. Leipzig, 1838. 18l.

—— et L. MANDL. Traité du microscope et de son emploie dans l'étude des corps organisés, suivi de recherches sur l'organisation des infusoires. 1 in-8, avec 14 planches. Paris, 1839. 8s.

ENCYCLOPEDIE Anatomique, comprenant l'anatomie descriptive, l'anatomie générale, l'anatomie pathologique, l'histoire du développement et celle des Races humaines, par MM. les professeurs S. Th. Bischoff, J. Henle, E. Huschke, S. Th. Sœmmerring, F. G. Theile, G. Valentin, J. Vogel, R. Wagner, G. et E. Weber, traduit de l'Allemand par A. J. L. Jourdan, membre de l'académie royale de médecine. 10 vol. in-8, fig. Prix de chaque, 7s. 6d.

Les tomes I., II., III., IV., V., VII., sont en vente. Il paraîtra 2 vol. tous les quatre mois.

Cet important ouvrage sera publié en neuf parties, ainsi divisée :—

1°. Biographie de Sœmmering, et histoire de l'anatomie et de la physiologie depuis Haller, par R. Wagner. 1 vol. in-8.

2°. Ostéologie et Syndesmologie, par S. T. Sœmmerring et R. Wagner.—Mécanique des mouvemens de l'homme, par O. et E. Weber. 1 vol. in-8, fig.

3°. Myologie et angéologie, par F. W. Theile. 1 vol. in-8.

4°. Névrologie et anatomie du cerveau, par Valentin. 1 vol. in-8, fig.

5°. Splanchnologie et organes des sens, par S. T. Sœmmerring et E. Huschke. 1 vol. in-8.

6°. Anatomie générale, ou histoire des tissus et de la composition chimique du corps humain, par Henle. 2 vol. in-8, fig.

7°. Histoire du développement de l'homme, par Bischoff. 1 vol. in-8, fig.

8°. Anatomie pathologique, par J. Vogel. 1 vol. in-8.

9°. Anatomie des races humaines et des nations, avec l'anatomie des téguments extérieurs, par R. Wagner. 1 vol. in-8.

EHRENBERG. Der Charakter und die Bestimmung des Mannes. 2 vols. 18mo. Wien, 1835. 4s.

EICHWALD. Plantarum Novarum vel minus Cognitarum. Vilnæ, 1831. Folio, 40 plates. 2l. 10s.

—— Fauna Caspio-Caucasia Nonnullis Observationibus Novis. Folio, with 40 coloured illustrations. Petropoli, 1841. 4l.

EISELT. Geschichte Systematik und Literatur der Insectenkunde. 8vo. Leipsig, 1836. 6s. 6d.

ELLIOTSON (J.) Numerous Cases of Surgical Operations without Pain in the Mesmeric State; with Remarks upon the Opposition of many Members of the Royal Medical and Chirurgical Society and others to the reception of the inestimable blessings of Mesmerism. 8vo. 1843. 2s. 6d.

See Teste, Zoist.

—— A Fine Portrait of Doctor. Engraved on Stone. London, 1844. 4s. 6d.

ENDLICHER. Genera Plantarum secundum ordines naturales disposita, and supplementary part. 4to. Vindobonæ, 1842-44. 6l.

—— und UNGER. Grundzüge der Botanik, with wood-cuts. 8vo. Wien, 1843. 16s.

—— Enchiridion Botanicum exhibens classes et ordines Plantarum. 8vo. Leipsig, 1841. 18s.

—— Die Medicinal-Pflanzen. 8vo. Wien, 1842. 13s.

ENGLEDUE. Cerebral Physiology and Materialism. With the result of the application of *Animal Magnetism* to the Cerebral Organs. With a Letter from Dr. Elliotson on Mesmeric Phrenology and Materialism. 8vo. London, 1842. 1s.

See Zoist.

EPPS. Domestic Homœopathy, or Rules for the Domestic Treatment of the Maladies of Infants, Children, and Adults, and for the Conduct and the Treatment during Pregnancy, Confinement, and Suckling. 1 vol. 18mo. 1841. 4s. 6d.

ERDMANN. Journal für praktische Chemie. From the commencement in 1828 to 1842. 42 vols. 8vo. bds. 24l.

ERESII Historia Plantarum. Cum adnotatione critica edidit F. Wimmer. 8vo. Vratislaviæ, 1842. 12s.

ERICHSON. Bericht über die Wissenschaftlichen Leistungen im Gebiete der Entomologie während des Jahres, 1842. 8vo. Berlin, 1844. 4s.

—— Genera et Species Staphylinorum, Insectorum, Coleopterorum familiæ. 8vo. Berolini, 1840. 1l. 10s.

ERNST et ENGRAMELLE. Papillons de l'Europe, peints d'après nature. 8 vol. in-4, avec 250 planches coloriées. Paris, 1769-91. 15l.

ERSCH UND GRUBER. Allgemeine Encyclopädie der Wissenschaften und Künste in alphabetischer Folge von gesammten Schriftstellern bearbeitet, mit Kupf. und Charten. 4to. Sectio I. Vol. I.-XXVIII. Leipsig, 1834. 16l. 8s.
     Sectio II. Vol. I.-XII. Leipsig, 1841. 9l. 12s.
     Sectio III. Vol. I.-X. Leipsig, 1841. 8l.

ESPER (E. T. C.) Die Europäischen Schmetterlinge. 7 bde. 4to. mit 424 ill. Kupf. Erlangen, 1785-1804. 25l.

—— Die Ausländischen Schmetterlinge. 4to. mit 160 illum. Kupf. Erlangen, 1829. 10l.

—— (J. F.) Ausführliche Nachricht von Neuentdeckten Zoolithen unbekannter vierfüssiger Thiere, und denen sie enthaltenden so wie verschiedenen andern denkwürdigen Grüften der Obergebürg. Lande d. Marggrafthums Bayreuth. Folio, mit 14 illum. Kupf. Nürnberg, 1774. 16s.

ESQUIROL. Des maladies mentales considérées sous les rapports médical hygiénique et médico-légal. 2 forts vol. in-8, avec un atlas de 27 planches gravées. Paris, 1838. 1l.

—— Examen du projet de loi sur les Aliénés. 1 in-8. Paris, 1838. 1s.

EVERSMANN. Fauna Lepidopterologica Volgo-Uralensis. 8vo. Casani, 1844. 1l. 8s.

EVEREST (T. R.) A Popular View of Homœopathy, exhibiting the Present State of the Science. 2d edition, amended and much enlarged. 8vo. London, 1836. 6s.

EXPOSITION (Souvenir de l') des produits de l'industrie Française de 1839; reproduction exacte des principales Etoffes façonnées et imprimées, recueil composé de 350 dessins réunis en 50 feuilles coloriées avec soin. Folio. Paris, 1840. 5*l.* 5*s.*

FABRICII Systema Piscatorum. 8vo. Brunsvigæ, 1804. 8*s.*

—— Systema Antliatorum. 8vo. Brunsvigæ, 1805. 8*s.*

FAVRE. Observations sur les Diceras. In-4, avec 5 planches. Genève, 1843. 6*s.*

—— Considérations Géologiques sur le Mont Salève et sur les Terrains des environs de Genève. 4to. avec deux planches. Genève, 1844. 6*s.*

FERRARII. De Florum Cultura. Libri IV. with plates. 4to. Romæ, 1633. 4*s.* 6*d.*

FICINUS. Flora der Tegend um Dresden. 12mo. Dresden, 1821. 4*s.*

FIEBER. Entomologische Monographien. With 10 plates. 4to. Leipzig, 1844. 8*s.*

FIELDING AND GARDNER. Sertum Plantarum; or Drawings and Descriptions of rare and undescribed Plants, from the Author's herbarium. 1 vol. 8vo. of 75 plates. London, 1844. 1*l.* 1*s.*

FLOGEL (Dr. J.) Compendium der Physiologie des Menschen. 8vo. Salzburg, 1840. 6*s.*

FLORE MEDICALE. Décrite par F. P. CHAUMENTON, D.M. peinte par TURPIN. 8 vol. in-8, boards, with coloured plates each. Paris, 1824. 6*l.*

FLOURENS. Anatomie générale de la Peau et des Membranes Muqueuses. In-4, avec 6 planches. Paris, 1843. 1*l.*

—— Mémoires d'Anatomie et de Physiologie comparées; accompagnées de huit planches. In-4. Paris, 1844. 18*s.*

—— Buffon, Histoire de ses Travaux et de ses Idées. In-12. Paris, 1844. 4*s.*

FODERE. Traité de Médecine légale et d'Hygiène publique, ou de police de santé. 6 vol. in-8. Paris, 1813. 1*l.* 10*s.*

FOLDI. L'Omeopatia Smascherata. 8vo. Milano, 1841. 3*s.* 6*d.*

FORSTER (H.) Praktische Anleitung zur Kenntniss der Gesetzgebung über Besteuerung des Branntweins und des Braumalzes. 8vo. with 41 plates. Berlin, 1830. 8*s.*

FOURNEL. Etude des Gîtes, Houillers, et Metallifères du Boccage Vendéen, faite en 1834 et 1835. Paris, 1836. 4to. and atlas fol. 18*s.*

FOVILLE. Traité complet de l'Anatomie, de la Physiologie, et de la Pathologie du Système Nerveux Cérébro-Spinal. Première partie. In-8, avec un atlas de 23 planches in-4. Paris, 1844. 1*l.* 8*s.*

FOY. Manuel d'hygiène, ou histoire des moyens propres à conserver la santé et à perfectionner le physique et le moral de l'homme. In-12. Paris, 1845. 4*s.* 6*d.*

FRANCOIS. Essai sur les convulsions Idcopathiques de la face. In-8. Bruxelles, 1843. 2*s.* 6*d.*

FRANK. De Curandis Hominum morbis Epitome prælectionibus Academicis dicata. 5 vols. 12mo. Mediolani, 1832. 1*l.* 5*s.*

—— (J. P.) Delectus Opusculorum Medicorum antehac in Germaniæ diversis academiis editorum. 3 vols. post 8vo. half-bound. Lipsiæ, 1790. 15*s.*

—— (F.S.) Verzeichniss der Münzen und Medaillen sammlung. 8vo. Wien, 1844. 2*s.* 6*d.*

FRIEDBERG. Die angebornen Krankheiten des Herzens und der grossen, Gefässe des Menschen. 8vo. Leipzig, 1844. 4*s.*

FRIES (E.) Systema Mycologicum, 2 vols. 8vo. Gryphiswaldæ, 1828. 12*s.*

—— Sind die Naturwissenschaften ein Bildungsmittel. 8vo. Dresden, 1844. 2*s.*

FREISLEBEN (J. C.) Die Sächsischen Erzgänge in einer Aufstellung ihrer Formationen. 8vo. Freiberg, 1843. 3*s.*

FUESSLINS. Verzeichnis der ihm bekannten Schweitzenschen Insecten. 4to. with one coloured plate. Zurich, 1775. 4*s.*

FURNIVALL. On the successful Treatment and Prevention of Consumption and Scrofula; female disorders connected therewith, strumous glandular swellings. 12mo. London, 1844. 6*s.*

FUSS. Correspondance Mathématique et Physique de quelques Célèbres Géomètres du XVIII. siècle. 2 vols. grand 8vo. St. Petersburg, 1843. 1*l.* 16*s.*

GALL ET SPURZHEIM. Recherches sur le système nerveux en général, et sur celui du Cerveau en particulier. In-4, avec une planche. Paris, 1809. 14*s.*

GARNIER ET HAREL. Des Falsifications des substances Alimentaires. In-12. Paris, 1844. 4*s.* 6*d.*

GAUDICHAUD. Recherches Générales sur l'Organographie, la Physiologie et l'Organogénie des Végétaux. 4to. with 18 coloured plates. Paris, 1840. 28*s.*

GAUTHIER (A.) Histoire du Somnambulisme. 2 vols. 8vo. Paris, 1842. 10*s.*

—— Introduction au Magnétisme. In-8. Paris, 1840. 7*s.*

—— Recherches historiques sur l'exercise de la médecine, dans les temples chez les peuples de l'antiquité. 12mo. Paris, 1844. 3*s.* 6*d.*

GAY-LUSSAC, a fine Portrait of. Folio. 3*s.* 6*d.*

GAZOLA. Ittiolitologia Veronese del Museo Bozziano, with 76 plates. Large folio. Verona, 1796. 5*l.*

GERBER AND GULLIVER. Elements of the General and Minute Anatomy of Man and the Mammalia, chiefly after Original Researches. To which is added an Appendix, comprising Researches on the Anatomy of the Blood, Chyle, Lymph, Thymous Fluid, Tubercle, &c. In 1 vol. 8vo. Text, and an Atlas of 34 Plates, engraved by L. ALDOUS. 2 vols. 8vo. Cloth boards, 1842. 1*l.* 4*s.*

GERHARDT. Précis de chimie organique. Tome premier. 8vo. Paris, 1844. 9*s.*

GESNERI Opera Botanica, edit. D. C. C. SCHMIDEL. 2 vols. folio, coloured plates. Nurenberg, 1751-71. 3*l.*

—— Tabulæ Phytographicæ analysin generum plantarum exhibentes cum commentatione. Edit. C. S. SCHING. Folio, avec 31 planches. Turici, 1795. 27*s.*

GIROD-CHANTRAS. Recherches Chimiques et Microscopiques sur les Conferves, Bisses tremelles. Avec 36 planches coloriées. In-4. Paris, 1802. 1*l.*

GLEICHEN. Observations Microscopiques sur les parties de la génération des plantes renfermées dans les fleurs. In-fol. avec 30 planches coloriées. Nuremberg, 1790. 2*l.*

GMELIN (J. F.) Enumeratio Stirpium agro Tubingensi indigenarum. 8vo. Tubingæ. 2*s.*

—— Flora Sibirica, sive historia Plantarum Sibiriæ. 4 vols. 4to. and atlas of plates bound. Petropoli, 1747-59. 2*l.*

—— Historia Fucorum. 4to. with 33 plates. Petropoli, 1768. 6*s.*

—— Reise durch Russland zur Untersuchung der drei Natur-Reiche. 4 vols. 4to. and numerous plates. St. Petersburg, 1770-84. 2*l.*

—— (LEOPOLD.) Handbuch der Chemie. 8vo. 18 numbers. Heidelberg, 1844. 1*l.* 18*s.*

GOEBEL (FR.) Pharmaceutische Waarenkunde. 2 vols. 4to. with 71 coloured plates. Eisenach, 1827-34. 4*l.* 4*s.*

GOEZE (J. A. E.) Versuch einer Naturgeschichte der Eingeweidewürmer thierischer Körper. 4to. with 44 plates. Leipzig, 1787. 1*l.* 5*s.*

—— Europaische Fauna oder Naturgeschichte der Europaischen Thiere. 9 vols. 8vo. Leipzig, 1791. 2*l.* 10*s.*

GOLDFUSS. Die Petrefakten Deutschlands und der angränzenden Länder. Mit 199 lithograph. Tafeln. 3 vols. fol. Düsseldorf, 1826-44. 18*l.* *Ouvrage complet.*

GRAHAM (T.) Elements of Chemistry; including the Application of the Science in the Arts. 1 thick vol. 8vo. illustrated with woodcuts, cloth boards. 1842. 1*l.* 6*s.* Part VI. and last containing Organic Chemistry, 8vo. 9*s.*

8   *H. Baillière, 219 Regent Street.*

GRABOWSKI. Flora von Oberschlesien, und dem Gesenke. 8vo. Breslau, 1843. 6s.

GRANT (Robt. E.) General View of the Distribution of Extinct Animals. 18mo. In the British Annual, 1839. London, 1829. 3s. 6d.

—— On the Present State of the Medical Profession in England; being the Annual Oration delivered before the Members of the British Medical Association, on the 21st of October, 1841. 2s. 6d.

—— On the Principles of Classification as applied to the Primary Divisions of the Animal Kingdom. 18mo. illustrated with 28 woodcuts. London, 1838. 3s. 6d. In the British Annual, 1838.

—— Outlines of comparative Anatomy. 8vo. Illustrated with 148 woodcuts. London, 1835—41. In boards, 1l. 8s. Part VII. with Title-page, just out, 1s. 6d.

GRAVENHORST. Ichneumonologia Eurpoœa. 3 vols. 8vo. Vratislaviæ, 1829. 2l. 15s.

GRISEBACH. Genera et Species Gentianarum adjectis Observationibus quibusdam Phytogeographicis. 8vo. Stuttgartiæ, 1839. 7s.

GRISOLLE (A.) Traité élémentaire et pratique de pathologie interne. 2 vol. in-8. Paris, 1844. 16s.

GROHMANN. Das Pest-Contagium in Egypten und Seine Quelle nebst einem Beitrage zum absperr-Systema. 8vo. Wien, 1844. 9s.

GUERIN. Iconographie du règne animal de G. Cuvier, ou représentation d'après nature de l'une des espèces le plus rémarquables, et souvent non encore figurée de chaque genre d'animaux, ouvrage pouvant servir d'atlas à tous les traités de zoologie, par F. E. Guerin, membre de diverses sociétés savantes nationales et étrangères. Paris, 1830-1844. 7 vol. grand in-8. Ce bel ouvrage est complet. Il a été publié en 50 livraisons, chacune de 10 planches gravées, et 2 vol. 8vo. de texte. Prix de chaque livraison, in-8, figures noires, 6s.

—— Le même, in-8, fig. col. 15s.

—— Le même, in-4, fig. col. 1l.

L'ouvrage complet est composé de 450 planches, avec un texte explicatif pour chacune des divisions qui se vendent séparément in-8, savoir :

	pl.	fig. n.	fig. col.
1°. Mammifères, avec le portrait de G. Cuvier	53	1 12	4 0
2°. Oiseaux	70	2 2	5
3°. Reptiles	39	0 18	2 5
4°. Poissons	70	2 2	5 5
5°. Mollusques et zoophytes	63	1 18	4 15
6°. Annélides, crustacés, et arachnides	53	1 12	4 0
7°. Insectes, avec le portrait de Latreille	111	3 6	8 5

—— Iconographie du règne animale de Cuvier. Livraisons 46 à 50, texte. 2 vols. 8vo. Paris, 1844. 1l. 10s.

—— et PECHERON. Genera des Insectes, ou exposition detaillée de tous les caractères propres à chacun des genres de cette classe d'animaux. In-8, avec grand nombre de planches coloriées. Paris, 1835. 1l. 16s.

GUILLOT (N.) Exposition anatomique de l'organisation du centre nerveux dans les quatres classes d'animaux vertébrés. In-4, with 18 plates. Paris, 1844. 14s.

GUIMPEL, WILDENOW, et HAYNE. Abildung der Deutschen Holzarten fur Forstmänner und Liebhaber der Botanik. 2 vols. 4to. with 216 coloured engravings. Berlin, 1815. 5l.

GULLIVER. See Gerber.

GUNTHER (G. B.) Die Verrenkung des ersten Daumengliedes nach der Rückenfläche. 4to. with 6 plates. Leipsig, 1844. 10s.

—— Die chirurgische anatomie in Abbildungen. Ein Handbuch für Studirende und Ausübende Aerzte, Wundärste, &c. 4to. avec 25 planches. Hamburgh, 1844. 16s.

GURLT (E. F.) Lehrbuch der vergleichenden Physiologie der Haus-Säugethiere. 8vo. with 3 plates. Berlin, 1837. 10s.

—— Handbuch der Vergleichenden Anatomie der Haus-Säugethiere. 2 vols. 8vo. Berlin, 1833. 18s.

GURLT (E. F.) Text zu den Anatomischen Abbildungen der Haus-Säugethiere. 8vo. Berlin, 1829. 8s.

—— Anatomie Abbildungen des Haus-Säugethiere. Second edition. Parts I.—XIV. Folio. Berlin, 1842—44. 6l. 6s.

GYNÆCIORUM Physicus et Chirurgicus, sive de Mulierum Affectibus Commentarii. 4 vols. 4to. in 2. Basilæ, 1576—1688. 2l.

HAENKE. Reliquiæ Haenkeanæ, seu Descriptiones et Icones Plantarum quas in America Meridionali et Boreali, in Insulis Phillipinis et Marianis collegit. Fasc. 1. Folio, 12 plates. Prague, 1825. 1l.

HAHN et W. HERRICH SCHAFFER. Die Wanzenartigen Insecten. Publié par livraison de 1 feuille de texte et 6 pl. in-8, col. Nuremberg, 1831—44. Prix de la liv. 4s.

43 livraisons sont en vente.

—— et C. L. KOCH. Die arachniden. Publié par livraisons de 1 feuille de texte et 6 pl. in-8, col. Nuremberg, 1831—44. Prix de la livraison, 4s.

60 livraisons sont en vente.

HAHNEMANN. Defence of Hahnemann and his Doctrines; including an Exposure of Dr. Alex. Wood's Homœopathy unmasked. 8vo. of 92 pages. London, 1844. 2s.

—— (S.) Organon der Heilkunst. 8vo. half-bound, with portrait. Leipsig. 8s.

HALL (Marshall). New Memoir on the Nervous System, True Spinal Marrow, and its Anatomy, Physiology, Pathology, and Therapeutics. 4to. with 5 engraved plates. London, 1843. 1l.

—— On the Diseases and Derangements of the Nervous System, in their Primary Forms and in their Modifications by Age, Sex, Constitution, Hereditary Predisposition, Excesses, General Disorder, and Organic Disease. 8vo. with 8 pl. engraved. London, 1841. 15s.

—— On the Mutual Relations between Anatomy, Physiology, Pathology, and Therapeutics, and the Practice of Medicine; being the Gulstonian Lectures for 1842. 8vo. with two coloured pl. and one plain. London, 1842. 5s.

As an Appendix to the above work.

HALLER. Historia Stirpium indigenarum Helvetiæ inchoata. 3 vols. folio, plates with Letters and Autographs from J. Hutton, Jain, J. E. Smith, and A. Haller. Bernæ, 1768. 2l.

—— Enumeratio Helvetiæ indigenarum. Folio. Gottingæ, 1762. 15s.

HANDBUCH der Speciellen Pathologie und Therapie der Acuten Krankheiten. Vol. I. 8vo. Berlin, 1844. 10s.

HARTMANN (Ph. Corr.) Institutiones Medico-Practicæ. 8vo. Part I. de Febribus. Viennæ, 1843. 8s.

—— Homœopathische Pharmacopæ. 8vo. Leipsig, 1834. 3s. 6d.

—— Theoriæ Morbi seu Pathologia Generalis. 8vo. Vindobonæ, 1840. 14s.

HASE. Uebersichttafeln zur Geschichte der Neueren Kunst. Folio. Dresden, 1827. 4s.

HAUSER. Versuch einer Pathologisch-Therapeutischen Darstellung des Schwammes der harten Hirnhaut und der Schädelknochen. 8vo. with 6 plates. Olmür, 1843. 3s. 6d.

HAYNE et DREVES. Choix de Plantes d'Europe. 5 vols. in-4, avec 125 planches coloriées. Leipsig, 1802. 2l.

—— Termini Botanici iconibus illustrati, oder botanische Kuntsprache durch Abbildungen erläutert. 69 pl. 4to. col. Berlin, 1807. 1l. 1s.

HAYNE, BRANDT, et RATZEBURG. Getreue Darstellung und Beschreibung der Arzneykunde Gebräuchlichen Gewächse. 13 vols. 4to. with 600 col. pl. Berlin, 1805-33. 15l. 15s.

HEDWIG. Filicum Genera et Species recentiore methodo accommodatæ analytice descriptæ. Folio, with 6 col. pl. Lipsiæ, 1769. 8s.

—— (R. A.) Observationum botanicarum, fasciculus primus. 4to. Lipsiæ. 1s.

—— Tremella nostoch. 4to. Lipsiæ. 1s. 6d.

HEDWIG. De Fibræ vegetabilis et Animalis ortu. Sect. I. 4to. Lipsiæ. 2s.
—— Species Muscorum frondosorum. 77 coloured plates. 4to. Lipsiæ, 1801. 3l. 2s.
—— Descriptio et Adumbratio Microscopico-Analytica Muscorum frondosorum. 4 vols. folio. with 160 coloured plates. 1782. 8l.
—— Fundamentum Historiæ Naturalis Muscorum frondosorum. 2 vols. 4to. tab. 20 ill. Lipsiæ, 1787–92. 1l. 2s.
—— Microskopisch - Analytische Beschreibungen und Abbildungen neuer und zweifelhafter Laub-Moose. Vol. IV. Folio, 40 coloured plates. 1l.
HEGER (A.) Erfahrungen im Gebiethe der Heilkunde. 12mo. Wien, 1842. 5s. 6d.
HEINE. Medicinisch-Topographische Skizze von St. Petersburgh. 4to. St. Petersburgh, 1844. 2s.
HELL (Xavier Hommaire de). Les Steppes de la Mer Caspienne, le Caucase, la Crimée, et la Russie Méridionale, voyage pittoresque, historique, et scientifique. Vol. I. or 14 livraisons, 1 vol. in-8, et atlas fol. Paris, 1844. 3l.
HERBST (G.) Das Lymphyefäsysystem und seine verrichtung. 8vo. Göttingen, 1844. 7s.
HERZIG (W.) Das Medicinische Wien. 12mo. with a plan of Vienna. Wien, 1844. 6s.
HEUSINGER (C. F.) Recherches de pathologie comparée. 2 parts, 4to. Paris, 1844. 16s.
HILPERT (J. L.) Englisch - Deutsches und Deutsch-Englisches Wörterbuch. 2 vols. 4to. in 4 parts. Carlsruhe, 1831. 2l. 2s.
HIMLY. Die Krankheiten und Missbildungen des menschlichen Anges und deren Heilung. 2 vols. 4to. mit 6 kupferfeln. Berlin, 1843. 2l. 10s.
HIPPOCRATE (Œuvres complètes d'). Traduction nouvelle, avec le texte Grec en regard, collationné sur les manuscrits et toutes les éditions; accompagnées d'une introduction, de commentaires médicaux, de variantes et de notes philologiques; suivi d'une table générale des matières, par E. Littrè, membre de l'Institut. Paris, 1839–44. Cet ouvrage formera environ 8 forts vol. in-8, de 600 à 700 pages chacun. Prix de chaque volume, 10s.
—— Il a été tiré quelques exemplaires sur Jésus-vélin. Prix de chaque volume, 1l.
Les tomes 1 à 4 sont vente.
HISINGER. Anteckningar I. Physik och Geogrosi under resor uti Sverige och Norrige. 2 vol. 8vo. with plates. Upsola, 1819. 10s.
HOBLYN. A Dictionary of Terms used in Medicine and the Collateral Sciences. Second Edition. 8vo. London, 1844. 10s.
HOCHSTETTER. Popular Botanik. 2 vols. 8vo. bound in 1, with 22 coloured plates. 18s.
HOERING (G.) Ueber den Sitz und die Natur de Grauen Staares. 8vo. with pl. Heilbronn, 1844. 3s.
HOEVEN. Recherches sur l'histoire naturelle et l'anatomie des limules. Folio, avec 7 planches. Leyde, 1838. 18s.
HOFF. Höhen-Measung einiger orte und Berge Zwischen Gotha und Coburg. Folio with a coloured plate. Gotha, 1828. 5s.
HOFFMANN (Dr. G. F.) Descriptio et Adumbratio Plantarum e Classe Cryptogamica Linnæi quæ Lichenes dicuntur. 3 vols. folio, containing 72 coloured plates. Leipzig, 1790–1801. 2l. 10s.
—— Vegetabilia Cryptogama. 4to. with 8 plates. 1787. 3s. 6d.
—— KOCH, MULLER, LINZ. Entomologische Hefte, Enthaltend Beiträge zur Weitern Kenntniss und Aufklärung der Insektengeschichte. 8vo. with 3 coloured plates. Frankfurt, 1803. 5s. 6d.
HOLMSKJOLD. Beata ruris otia Fungis Danicis impensa. 4 vols. folio, with 42 coloured plates. Haunie, 1799. 15l.
HOOKER (Sir W. J.) Icones Plantarum, New Series. Vols. I. II. and III. containing each 100 plates with explanations. 8vo. cloth. London, 1842–44. 1l. 8s. each vol.
—— The London Journal of Botany. Vols. I. and II., with 24 plates each, boards. 1842-3. 1l. 10s. each vol.
Also published monthly, with 2 plates. Price 2s. 6d.

HOOKER (Sir W. J.) Notes on the Botany of the Antarctic Voyage conducted by Capt. Jas. Clark Ross, R.N., F.R.S., in H.M.S. *Erebus* and *Terror*, with Observations on the Tussac Grass of the Falkland Islands. 8vo. with 2 coloured plates. London, 1843. 4s.
HOPER. Flora der Graffchaft Schaumburg und der Umgegend. 8vo. Rinteln, 1838. 4s.
HORN (H.) Physico-Pathologische Darstellung des Schleimfiebers. 8vo. Augsberg, 1844. 6s.
HOST (N. T.) Flora Austriaca. 2 vols. 8vo. half-bound. Viennæ, 1827–31. 1l. 8s.
HUBENER. Die gastrischen Krankheiten monographisch dargestellt. 2 vols. 8vo. Leipzig, 1844. 16s.
HUFELAND. Manual of the Practice of Medicine, the Result of Fifty Years' Experience. By W. C. Hufeland, Physician to the late King of Prussia, Professor in the University of Berlin. From the Sixth German Edition. Translated by C. Beuchhausen and R. Nelson. 8vo. bound. London, 1844. 15s.
—— Am Tage seiner Jubel-Feier. Folio. Berlin 1833. 8s.
—— Journal der praktischen Heilkunde. 75 Bde. 1795–1833. 15l.
HULL (A. G.) The Homœopathic Examiner. Subscriptions for Vol. III. 1l. 10s. Vols. I. and II. each 1l. 10s. New York, 1839–40.
HUMBOLDT (A.) Sur les lois que l'on observe dans la distribution des formes végétales. 8vo. Paris, 1816. 2s.
HUNTER (Dr. W.) The Anatomy of the Human Gravid Uterus, exhibited in 31 figures. Atlas, fol. 1774. 4l. 4s.
HUTER (K. C.) Lehrbuch der Geburtshülfe für Hebammen. Second edition. 8vo. Leipzig, 1844. 6s.

JABLONSKY und HERBST. Natur System aller bekannten In-und Ausländischen Insecten, Schmetterlinge und Käfer. 21 vols. 8vo. half-bound, and 3 atlases containing 539 pl. 4to. beautifully coloured. Berlin, 1783–1801. 21l.
JACQUEMONT (Victor). Voyage dans l'Inde pendant les Années 1828 à 1832. Publié sous les auspices de M. Guizot. 49 livraisons 4to. contenant 246 planches. Paris, 1840–44. Prix de chaque, 8s. "*Presque toutes les planches sont relatives à la Botanique des Indes.*"
JACQUIN. Hortus botanicus Vendobonensis. Vol. III. folio, with 100 coloured plates. 1l. 1s.
—— Selectarum Stirpium Americanarum historia, 12mo. Manhemii, 1798. 3s. 6d.
—— Miscellanea Austriaca ad Botanicum, Chemiam et Historiam naturalem Spectantia, cum figuris partim Coloratis. 2 vols. 4to. 1778. 15s.
—— Collectanea ad Botanicum, Chemiam, Historiam naturalem Spectantia, cum figuris, 4 vols. et Suppl. 4to. 1786-96. 8l.
JAHN (G. A.) Geschichte der Astronomie. Vol. I. 8vo. Leipzig, 1844. 16s.
JAHR (G. H. G.) New Homœopathic Pharmacopœia and Posology; or the Preparations of Homœopathic Medicines, and the Administration of Doses, with Additions, by James Kitchen, M.D. 8vo. Philadelphia, 1842. 12s.
—— Systematisch-alphabetisches repertorium der Homoopathischer Arzneimittellehre. Vols. I. and II. Vol. III. part I. 8vo. Düsseldorf, 1844. 2l. 2s.
—— New Manual of Homœopathic Medicine, from the third original edition, with Notes and Preface by Dr. P. Curie and Dr. Laurie. In 2 vols. post 8vo. 1841. 1l. 8s
See Curie, Laurie.
—— Elementary Notices on Homœopathy, translated by Gilioli, M.D. Second edition. 18mo. London, 1845. 3s.
JAHRBUCH Berlinisches für die Pharmacie, Von V. Rose, Gehlen, Döbereiner, Kastner, Stolze, Meissner, V. Lucæ, und Lindes. 1795–1840. 12mo. Berlin. In all, 45 years. Half-bound, 9l.
JAMAIN (M. A.) Manuel de petite Chirurgie. In-12. Paris, 1844. 3s. 6d.

JAMESON. Remarks on Vivisection, in a Letter to the Earl of Caernarvon, President of the Society for preventing Cruelty to Animals. 1s. 6d.

JANSON. Mélanges de chirurgie et comptes rendus de la pratique chirurgicale de l'Hôtel Dieu de Lyon. In-8. Paris, 1844. 7s.

JENNERI Disquisitio de Caussis et Affectibus Variolarum Vaccinarum. 4to. with 4 coloured plates. Vindobonæ 1799. 5s. 6d.

JENTI (C. N.) Demonstratio Uteri. Atlas fol. with plates on boards. Nürnberg, 1761. 1l. 1s.

ILLIGER. Magazin für Insektenkunde. 4 vols. bd. in 2. Braunschweig, 1801-5. 1l. 8s.

IORG. Handbuch der Krankheiten des Weibers. 8vo. with 4 plates. Reutlingen, 1832. 14s.

KAAN. Psychopathia sexualis. 8vo. Lipsiæ, 1844. 3s.

KAEMTZ. Complete Course of Meteorology, with Notes by Ch. Martins, and an Appendix by E. Lalanne. Translated, with Notes, by C. V. Walker. Illustrated with 15 plates. London, 1845. 12s. 6d.

KARSTNER (R. W. G.) Archiv für die gesammte Naturlehre. 19 vols. 8vo. Nürnberg, 1824-30.— Archiv für Chemie und Meteorologie. 9 vols. 8vo. Nürnberg, 1830-35. Le tout, 6l.

KARSTEN (G.) Imponderabilium præsertim Electricitatis theoria Dynamica. 4to. with 2 coloured plates. Berolini, 1843. 2s. 6d.

—— (C. J. B.) Philosophie der Chemie. 8vo. Berlin, 1843. 6s.

KASTNER (A. G.) Neue Abhandlungen aus der Naturlehre, Haushaltungskunst und Mechanik von der Schwedischen Academie der Wissenschaften. 12 vols. 8vo. with plates. Leipzig, 1784-92. 1l. 1s.

KAUP (J. J.) Classification der Säugethiere und Vögel. 8vo. with 2 plates. Darmstadt, 1844. 4s.

—— Description d'ossemens fossiles de mammifères inconnus jusqu'à présent, qui se trouvent au Museum de Darmstadt. 4to. and atlas folio. Darmstadt, 1839. 5l. 8s.

KEFERSTEN. Teutschland Geognostisch Geologisch dargestellt. Mit charten und durchschnittszeichnungen. 7 bde. 8vo. und kupf. Weimar, 1821-32. 4l. 4s.

KERNER. Le Raisin. Ses espèces et variétés dessinées et coloriées d'après nature, en 12 livraisons, avec 144 dessins original. Large folio, morocco gilt, gilt edges. Stuttgart, 1803-15. 40l.

KILIAN. Atlas of Midwifery. Published in 80 plates, grand folio. Düsseldorf, 1835-40. Complete work. 4l. 4s.

KLEIN (J. T.) Sammlung verschiedener Vögel Eier in natürlicher Grösse und mit lebendigen Farben geschildert und beschrieben. 4to. with 21 coloured plates. Leipzig, 1766. 16s.

—— Ova Avium Plurimarum ad Naturalem Magnitudinem Delineata, et Genuinis Coloribus picta (Latin and German). 4to. with 21 coloured plates. Leipzig, 1766. 16s.

—— Naturalis Dispositio Echinodermatum. 2 vols. 4to. with 54 fine plates. Lipsiæ. 1l. 15s.

—— Specimen Descriptionis Petrefactorum Gedanensium. 4to. with 24 plates. Nurenberg, 1770. 2l.

—— Historia Piscium Naturalis. 4to. avec des planches. Gedani, 1740. 10s.

—— Naturalis Dispositio Echinodermatum accessit Lucubratiuncula de Oculeis Echinorum Marinorum cum Spicilegio de Belemnitis. Gedani, 1734. 15s.

—— Zum Medaillen und Münzcopiren. 12mo. with plates. 1754. 2s. 6d.

KLENCKE. Mémoire en réponse à la question suivante, donner l'histoire ; les propriétés physiques et chimiques, le mode d'extraction de l'huile de foie de Morue et de Baliene (Ol. Jecoris, Aselli, et Ol. Ceti) ; faire connaitre comparativement et par des faits leur histoire thérapeutique. In-8. Anvers. 3s.

—— Zootomisches Taschenlexicon. 18mo. Leipzig, 1844. 7s.

—— (P. F. H.) Ueber die Contagiosität der Eingeweidewürmer. 8vo. Jena, 1844. 3s.

KLIEMSTEIN (J.) Dissertatio Inauguralis enumerans genera Coleopterorum in Dustschmia Fauna Austriæ. 4to. Lineth, 1817. 1s. 6d.

KLINISCHE Hand-Bibliothek : eine Auserlesene Sammlung der besten neuern Klinisch-Medicinischen Schriften des Auslandes. 6 bde. 8vo. Weimar, 1829-36. 1l. 10s.

KLUG (F.) Entomologiæ Brasilianæ. 4to. with 5 coloured plates. 5s.

—— Monographia Siricum Germaniæ. 4to. Cum Tabulis æneis coloratis viii. Berlin, 1803. 12s.

KNAUR (T.) Selectus Instrumentorum Chirurgicorum in usum Discentium et Practicorum. Folio, with 25 plates. Vienna, 1796. 8s.

KNIPE. Geological Map of the British Isles and part of France, shewing also the Inland Navigation by means of Rivers and Canals, the Railways and principal Roads, and Sites of the Minerals. Beautifully coloured. Size of the Map, 5 feet 4 inches by 4 feet 4 inches. London, 1843. Price, mounted on rollers, and varnished, 4l. 4s.; and ditto, in a case, 4l. 4s.

—— Geological Map of England and Wales. Third edition, beautifully coloured, mounted. London, 1841. 2l. 12s. 6d.

KNORR (G. W.) Vergnügen der Augen und des Gemüths, in Vorstellung einer allgem. Sammlung von Muscheln und andern Geschöpfen welche im Meer gefunden werden. With numerous coloured plates. 6 vols. 4to. Nürnberg, 1775. Bound. 8l.

—— Deliciæ Naturæ Selectæ, edent Muller. Fol. avec 73 col. pl. bound. Dordrecht, 1771. 8l.

—— Thesaurus Rei Herbariæ Hortensisque Universalis exhibens Figuras Florum, Herbarum, Arborum, Fruticum. 2 vols. fol. with 300 coloured plates. Witteberge, 1771. 4l.

KOCH (G. D. J.) Synopsis Floræ Germanicæ et Helveticæ. Second edition. Vol. I. 8vo. Leipzig, 1843. 12s. 6d.

—— (E. J.) Die Mineral-quellen Deutschlands und der Schweiz. 8vo. Wien, 1844. 3s. 6d.

KONINCK. Description des Animaux fossiles qui se trouvent dans le Terrain Houiller, et dans le système supérieur du Terrain Anthraxifère de la Belgique. In-4. Planches, 12 livraisons. Liege, 1844. 4l. 10s.

KOPP. Dentürerdigkeiten in der ärztlichen Praxis. Vol. V. 8vo. Frankfort, 1844. 10s.

KRAUSS. Die Südafrikanischen crustaceen eine Zusammenstellung aller Bekannten Malacastraca. 4to. with 4 plates. Stuttgart, 1843. 9s.

KREID. Magnetische und Meteorologische Beobachtungen zu Prag. 4to. Prag, 1843. 15s.

KROCKER. Flora Silesiaca, with coloured plates. 3 vols. Vratislaviæ, 1787. 1l. 10s.

KUNTH (K. S.) Pharmacopœa Borussica aufgeführten officinellen, Gewächse. 8vo. Berlin, 1834. 6s.

—— Flora Berolinensis. 2 vol. 8vo. Berlin, 1838. 1s.

—— Enumeratio Plantarum omnium hucusque Cognitarum secundum Familias Naturales disposita, adjectis Characteribus, Differentiis et Synonymis. 5 vol. 8vo. and plates. Stuttgardiæ, 1833-43. 3l. 15s.

KUNZE (G.) Supplemente der Riedgräser (Carices) zu Schkuhr's Monographie. Vol. I. Nos. 1, 2, 3, 8vo. with 20 coloured plates. Each part 8s. Leipzig, 1841-43.

KUPPRECHT (J. B.) Ueber das Chrysanthemum Indicum feine Geschichte Bestimmung und Pflege. 8vo. Wien, 1833. 4s.

KUTTNER. Medecinische Phænomenologie. Ein Handwörterbuch für die Ärztliche Praxis. 2 vols. 8vo. Leipzig, 1836. 1l.

KUTZING. Ueber die Verwandlung der Infusorien in niedere Algenformen avec 1 planche. 4to. Nordhausen, 1844. 3s.

LABILLARDIERE. Novæ Hollandiæ plantarum specimen. 2 vols. 4to. bound. Parisiis, 1804-5. 6l.

LACAUCHE. Etudes hydrotomiques et micrographiques. 8vo. avec 4 planches. Paris, 1844. 3s.

LAFITTE. Symptomatologie Homœopathique, ou tableau synoptique de toute la matière médicale pure. 7 liv. gd. 8vo. Paris, 1842-44. 1l. 15s.

LAFORE. Traité des maladies particulières aux grands ruminans, precédé de notions étendues sur l'amélioration et l'hygiène de ces animaux, suivi d'un traité sur les vaches laitières, avec une gravure. 8vo. Paris, 1843. 10s.

LALANNE. Meteorology. *See* KAEMTZ.

LAMARK (J. B. P.) Histoire naturelle des animaux sans vertèbres, présentant les caractères généraux et particuliers de ces animaux, leur distribution, leurs classes, leurs familles, leurs genres, et la citation synonymique des principales espèces qui s'y rapportent. Deuxième édition, revue et augmentée des faits nouveaux dont la science s'est enrichie jusqu'à ce jour, par M. G. P. DESHAYES et H. MILNE EDWARDS. XI. forts vol. in-8. Paris, 1836-44. Prix de chaque, 8s.

Les tomes I.-X. sont en vente.

LAMOUROUX. Corallina; or, a Classical Arrangement of Flexible Coralline Polypidoms, selected from the French, with 19 plates. 8vo. cloth. London, 1824. 8s.

LANGENBECK (C. J. M.) Nosologie und Therapie der chirurgischen Krankheiten. Vol. 1-5. 8vo. Göttingen, 1840. 2l.

—— De Retina Observationes Anatomico-pathologicæ. 4to. with 4 plates. Gottingæ, 1836. 7s.

LAURIE (T.) Homœopathic Domestic Medicine. 12mo. 2d edition. London, 1844. 8s.

LAVACHERIE. De la gangrène de la bouche, avec nécrose des os maxillaires. 8vo. 1s. 6d.

LEBAUDY. The Anatomy of the Regions interested in the Surgical Operations performed upon the Human Body; with occasional Views of the Pathological Conditions which render the interference of the Surgeon necessary. In a series of 18 plates on India paper, the size of life. With additions. Folio. London, 1835. 1l. 4s.

LE BLANC. Nouvelle méthode d'opérer les hernies, avec une essai sur les hernies rares et peu connues, par M. HOIN. 3 vol. in-8. Paris, 1782. 12s.

LECOQ (H.) Precis élémentaire de Botanique et de Physiologie végétale, contenant l'Histoire complète de toutes les parties des Plantes, et l'Exposition des règles à suivre pour décrire et classer des Végétaux. In-8. Paris, 1831. 5s.

—— ET JUILLET. Nouveau Dictionnaire Raisonné des Termes de Botanique et des Familles naturelles, contenant l'Etymologie et la Description détaillée de tous les Organes, leur Synonomie, et de la Définition des Adjectifs. 1 vol. in-8. Paris, 1841. 9s.

LEDEBOUR. Flora Altaica. 4 vols. bound, and Supplement. Berolini, 1829-36. 1l. 10s.

LEDRU (ANDRÉ PIERRE). Voyage aux Iles de Ténériffe, La Trinité, St. Thomas, St. Croix, et Porto Ricco. 2 vol. in-8. Paris, 1810. 8s.

LEE (R.) The Anatomy of the Nerves of the Uterus. Folio, with 2 engraved plates. London, 1841. 8s.

LEERS (J. D.) Flora Herbornensis exhibans Plantas circa Herbornam Nassoviorum crescentes. 8vo. with 16 plates. Berlin, 1789. 8s.

LEHMANN. Lehrbuch der Physiologischen Chemie. 8vo. Leipzig, 1842. 9s.

LEIBNITII ET BERNOULLII. Commercium Philosophicum et Mathematicum. 2 vols. 4to. Lausanne, 1745. 15s.

LEIGHTON (W. A.) A Flora of Shropshire. 8vo. cloth, with plates. London, 1841. 18s.

LE MAOUT (E.) Leçons élémentaires de Botanique, fondées sur l'analyse de 50 plantes vulgaires, et formant un traité complet d'Organographie et de Physiologie Végétale, à l'usage des étudiens et des gens du monde. In-8, avec 254 figures. Paris, 1843. Prix, figures noires, 15s.; coloriées, 1l. 5s.

LEMONNIER. Programme de l'enseignement de l'histoire naturelle dans les collèges, adopté par le conseil royal de l'instruction publique, disposé en 49 tableaux méthodiques. Troisième édit. in-4. Paris, 1840. Cartonné, fig. coloriées, 1l. 4s.; fig. noires, 10s.

LEONHARD. Propaedeutik der Mineralogie mit 10 schwarzen und ausgemalten Kupfertafeln. Folio. Frankfort, 1817. 1l. 4s.

LE PRIEUR. L'homme considéré dans ses rapports avec l'atmosphère, ou nouvelle doctrine des épidémies. 2 vol. in-8. Paris, 1825. 10s.

LEROY (D'ETIOLLES). Receuil de lettres et de mémoires adressés à l'Académie des Sciences pendant les années 1842 et 1843. In-8. Paris, 1844. 5s.

LERSCH (L.) Fabius Planciades Fulgentius de abstrusis Sermonibus. 8vo. Bonn, 1844. 4s.

LEVAILLANT (F.) Histoire naturelle des perroquets. 2 vols. large folio, demie rel. with 139 coloured plates. Paris, 1804. 12l.

LEVRET. Essai sur l'Abus des règles générales et contre les préjugés qui s'opposent au progrès de l'art des Accouchmens, avec figures. In-8. Paris, 1766. 4s.

—— Observations sur la cure radicale de plusieurs polypes de la Matrice de la Gorge, et du Nez. Troisième édition. 1 vol. in-8. Paris, 1759. 6s.

—— L'art des accouchemens, démontré par des principes de physique et de méchaniques. Troisième édition, revue et corrigée par l'Auteur; avec un abrégé de son sentiment sur les aphorismes de MAURICEAU. In-8. Paris, 1766. 5s.

LEVY (M.) Traité d'Hygiène publique et privée. Vol. I. In-8. Paris, 1844. 7s.

LEYSSER (F. W.) Flora Halensis exhibens plantas circa halam salicam crescentes secundum systema sexuale Linnæanum distributas. 8vo. Hale Salicæ, 1783. 4s.

L'HERITIER. Traité de chimie pathologique, ou recherches chimiques sur les solides et les liquides du corps humain, dans leurs rapports avec la physiologie et la pathologie. In-8, avec une pl. Paris, 1842. 9s.

—— Stirpes Novæ Descriptionibus et Iconibus illustratæ. Large fol. avec 84 planches. Paris, 1784. 1l. 10s.

—— Cornus Specimen Botanicum sistens Descriptiones et Icones specierum Corninus cognitarum. Folio, avec 6 planches. Paris, 1788. 10s.

LIEBIG. Poggendorff und Wholer Handwörterbuch der reinen und angewandten Chemie. Vol. I. 8vo. bd. Braunschweig, 1842. 18s.

—— Chemische Briefe. 12mo. Heidelberg, 1844.

—— Traité de Chimie Organique. 3 vols. 8vo. 6s. Paris, 1840-44. 1l. 5s.

—— Séparément. Vol. III. 8vo. Paris, 1844. 7s.

LINNÆI Amœnitates Academicæ. 10 vols. 8vo. plates. Editio tertia. Erlangæ, 1787. 2l. 5s.

—— Systema, Genera, Species Plantarum. Editio critica, adstricta, conferta sive Codex Botanicus Linnæanus, cum plena editionum discrepantia exhibens. In usum Botanicorum Practicum, edidit H. E. RICHTER. 4to. Lipsiæ, 1840. 3l. 16s.

—— Systema Vegetabilium. edent. SPRENGEL. 5 vols. 8vo. half-bound. Gottingæ, 1825. 3l. 10s.

—— Oratio de Necessitate Peregrinationum intra Patriam, &c. 8vo. Lugd. Bat. 1743. 1s. 6d.

—— Genera Plantarum. Editio nova curante C. SPRENGEL. 2 vols. 8vo. Gottingæ, 1832. 1l.

LINNÆA: ein Journal für die Botanik in ihrem ganzen Umfange Herausgegeben von SCHLECTENDAL. From the commencement, in 1826, to 1832. 13 vols. 8vo. boards. 9l.

LITTRE. Œuvres complètes d'Hippocrate, traduction nouvelle, avec le texte Grec en regard. Tome IV. In-8. Paris, 1844. 10s. Les quatres volumes, 2l.

—— Aphorismes d'Hippocrate. In-12. Paris, 1844. 3s.

LITZMANN (C. T. C.) Das kindbettfieber in nosologischer, geschichtlicher und therapeutischer Beziehung. 8vo. Halle, 1844. 12s.

LOHRMANN (W. G.) Topographie der sichtbaren Mondoberfläche. Part I. 4to. with 6 plates. Dresden, 1824. 15s.

—— Poids médicaux et pharmaceutiques de tous les états et villes libres de l'Europe, en 28 tableaux particuliers. In-4. Leipsic, 1832. 3s.

LOISELEUR-DESLONGCHAMPS. Flora Gallica, seu enumeratio Plantarum in Gallia sponte nascentium, secundum LINNÆUM disposita, addita familiarum naturalium synopsi. Nova editio, emendata, aucta. Parisiis, 1828. 2 vol. in-8, cum Tabulis XXXI. 16s.

LONGET (F. A.) Anatomie et physiologie du système nerveux de l'homme et des animaux vertébrés; ouvrage contenant des observations pathologiques relatives au système nerveux et des expériences sur les animaux des classes supérieures. 2 vol. in-8. Paris, 1842. 18s.

LOUREIRO (JOANNES). Flora Cochinchinensis, sistens plantas in regno Cochinchina nascentes. Edent. WILLDENOW. 8vo. 2 vols. in 1. Berlin, 1793.

LOW (G.) See BOUSSINGAULT.

LUDWIG (C. FR.) Delectus Opusculorum. Vol. I. 8vo. Leipzig, 1790. 6s.

—— (C. G.) Genera Plantarum. 8vo. Lipsiæ, 1760. 6s.

—— Scriptores nevrologici minores selecti. 81 Opera minora ad Anatomiam, Physiologiam, et Pathologiam, Nervorum spectantia. 4 vols. 4to. plates. Leipzig, 1791-95. 3l. 15s.

LUGOL. Recherches et observations sur les causes des maladies Scrofuleuses. In-8. Paris, 1844. 7s.

LYONET. Traité anatomique de la chenille qui ronge le bois de saule. In-4, avec 18 planches. La Haye, 1762. 2l. 10s.

MAGAZIN der Gesellschaft Naturforschender Freunde zu Berlin. Neue Schriften. 4 vols. 4to. containing 26 plates. Berlin, 1795-1803. 4l.

MAGAZINE of Zoology and Botany. Conducted by Sir W. JARDINE, Bart., P. J. SELBY, Esq., and Dr. JOHNSTON. 2 vols. 8vo. Edinburgh, 1837-38. 15s.

MAGNETISM (le), et le Somnambulism devant les corps savants la cour de Rome et les Théologiens. 8vo. Paris, 1844. 7s.

MAGNOL. Hortus Regius Monspeliensis. 8vo. 19 plates. 1697. 2s.

MAILLIOT. Traité Pratique de Percussier. 12mo. Paris, 1843. 3s. 6d.

MAN, Natural History of. See PRICHARD.

MANDL. Anatomie Microscopique, divisée en deux séries, tissus et organes, liquides. Paris, 1838-44. Cet ouvrage formera 25 livr., publiées par cahiers de 5 feuilles et de texte et 2 pl. Prix de chaque livraison, 6s.

16 livraisons publiées comprennent : Première série : 1º, *Muscles* ; 2º et 3º, *Nerfs et Cerveau* ; 4º et 5º, *Appendices tégumentaires* ; 6º, *Terminaison des nerfs* ; 7º, *Cartilages, Os et Dents* ; 8º, *Tissus celluleux et adipeux* ; 9º, *Tissus séreux, fibreux et élastiques*. Deuxième série : 1º, *Sang* ; 2º, *Pus et Mucus* ; 3º, *Lait et Urine, épidermes, et Epithelium, Glandes*.

—— Manuel d'anatomie générale appliquée à la physiologie et la pathologie. In-8, avec 5 pl. gr. Paris, 1843. 8s.

—— ET EHREMBERG (C. G.) Traité pratique du Microscope et de son emploi dans l'étude des corps organisés suivi de recherches sur l'organisation des animaux infusoires. In-8, avec 14 pl. Paris, 1830. 8s.

MANN (J. G.) Deutschlands gefährlichste Giftpflanzen. Tab. 24 coloured. Folio. Stuttgart, 1829. 1l.

MANUAL of Veterinary Homœopathy. Comprehending the Treatment of the Diseases in Domestic Animals. 18mo. London, 1841. 4s.

MAPPI. Historia Plantarum Asiaticarum. 4to. with 7 plates. Amstelodami, 1742. 3s.

MARCHAND. Lehrbuch der Physiologischen Chemie. 8vo. Berlin, 1844. 10s.

MARCHETTI. Dell' Ottalmoscopia e dell' Introduzione allo studio dell' ottalmologia. 8vo. Pavia, 1834. 6s.

MARSHAL. Des Abces Phlegmoneux intra pelviens. 8vo. Paris, 1844. 3s. 6d.

MARTIN (W. C. L.) A General Introduction to the Natural History of Mammiferous Animals. With a particular View of the Physical History of Man, and the more closely allied Genera of the Order "Quadrumana," or Monkeys. Illustrated with 296 Anatomical, Osteological, and other Engravings on Wood, and 12 full-plate Representations of Animals, drawn by W. HARVEY. 1 vol. 8vo. London, 1841. 16s.

MARTINI. Der verbesserte geschichte Haushalter und fertige Kauffmann. 8vo. Berlin, 1797. 2s. 6d.

—— UND CHEMNITZ. Neues systematiches Conchylien-Cabinet. 12 vol. in-4. Fig. col. Nürnberg, 1769-1820. 20l.

MARTINS (CH.) Meteorology. See KAEMTZ.

MARTIUS. Lehrbuch der pharmaceutischen Zoologie. 8vo. with 3 plates. Stuttgart, 1838. 6s.

—— Grundriss der Pharmakognosie des Pflanzenreichs. 8vo. Erlangen, 1832. 9s.

—— Systema materiæ medicæ vegetabilis Brasiliensis. 8vo. Lipsiæ, 1843. 4s.

—— (Ph.) Decas Plantarum Mycetoidearum. 4to. with a coloured plate. 2s.

—— Agrostographia Brasiliensis, auctore NEES ab ESSENBECK. 8vo. Stuttgartiæ, 1829. 12s.

—— Dissertatio Inauguralis sistens Plantarum Horti Academici Erlangensis Enumerationem. 8vo. Erlangen. 2s.

—— Choix des plantes rémarquables du Jardin Botanique Royal de Munic. In-4, avec 16 planches, fig. col. Franckfurt, 1827-31. 1l. 4s.

—— UND SPIX (J. B. von). Avium species novæ. Curâ J. B. de SPIX. 2 vols. 4to. cum 222 tabulis lith. et col. Munich, 1825-6. 33l. 12s.

—— Serpentum species novæ. Curâ J. WAGLER. Cum 26 tabulis lith. et col. Munich, 1824. 6l. 6s.

—— Testacea fluviatilia. Collegit et curavit J. B. de SPIX et J. A. WAGNER. Cum 29 tabulis lith. et col. Munich, 1827. 3l. 9s.

—— Genera et species Piscium. Curâ J. B. de SPIX et L. AGASSIZ. Cum 98 tabulis lith. et col. Munich, 1829-31. 14l. 12s.

—— Delectus Animalium articulatorum. Curâ M. PERTY. 3 Parts cum 40 tabulis lith. et col. Munich, 1830-34. 1l.

—— Reise in Brasilien in Jahr. 1817-20. 3 vols. 4to. and atlas of 53 lith. pls. folio. 8l. 12s.

—— Von Dem Rechtszustande unter Den Ureinwohnern Brasiliens. 4to. Munchen, 1832. 8s.

—— Icones Plantarum Cryptogamicarum auc. C. F. P. MARTIUS. Cum 76 tab. col. 4to. Monachii, 1827-34. 15l.

—— Genera et Species Palmarum, cur. C. F. P. MARTIUS. VI. fasc. cum 177 tab. col. Grand in-fol. Monachii, 1823-36. 60l.

—— Nova Genera et Species Plantarum, coll. et descr. C. F. P. MARTIUS et J. G. ZUCCARINI. 3 vols. 4to. cum 300 tab. col. Monachii, 1824-31. 50l.

—— UND ENDLICHER. Flora Brasiliensis sive Enumeratio Plantarum in Brasilia. Folio. Parts I. II. et III. avec 34 planches, fig. noires. Vindobonæ, 1840-41. 5l. 16s.

MARX. Ueber die Abnahme der Krankheiten durch die Zunahme der Civilisation. 4to. Göttingen, 1844. 3s.

—— (K. F. H.) Akesios Blicke in die ethischen Beziehungen der medicin. 8vo. Göttingen, 1844. 3s.

—— Eine Gedächtniss Rede, zum Andenken an JOHANN FRIEDRICH BLUMENBACH. 4to. Göttingen, 1840. 3s.

MATTEUCCI. Traité des Phénomènes Electro-Physiologique des Animaux suivi d'études Anatomique sur le système nerveux et sur l'organe électrique de la Torpille avec des planches. 8vo. Paris, 1844. 8s.

MATTHIOLI. Commentarii in sex Libros Pedacii Dioscoridis Anazarbei de Medica Materia. 2 vols. folio. Venetiis, 1565. 1l. 10s.

MAYER. Analecten für Vergleichen de anatomie. 4to. Mit. Sieben Tafeln. Bonn, 1835. 6s.

—— (J. C. A.) Einheimische Giftgewächse welche für Menschen am schädlichsten sind. Folio, with 11 coloured plates. 1796-1801, und Vorzügliche Einheimische Essbare Schwämme. Folio, with 3 coloured plates. Berlin, 1801. 15s.

MEADE (W.) A Manual for Students who are Preparing for Examination at Apothecaries Hall. 12mo. London, 1839. 10s. 6d.

MECKEL. De Duplicitate Monstrosa commentarius. Folio. Halæ, 1725. 1l.

MECKEL. System der vergleichenden Anatomie. 8 vols. 8vo. Halle, 1821. 3*l.*

—— Tabulæ Anatomico-Pathologicæ. Pt. I.-IV. mit 33 Kupf. Leipsig, 1817-26. 5*l.*

—— (F.) Manuel d'anatomie générale, descriptive et pathologique; traduit de l'Allemand, et augmentée des faits nouveaux dont la science s'est enrichie jusqu'à ce jour, par G. BRESCHET, et A. J. L. JOURDAN, D.M.P. 3 vol. in-8, de 800 pages chacun. Paris, 1825. 2*l.* 10*s.*

—— Traité général d'anatomie comparée; trad. de l'Allemand par RIESTER et A. SANSON. 10 vol. in-8. Paris, 1829-38. 3*l.*

—— Deutsches archiv für physiologie. 8 vol. in-8, fig. Halle, 1815-23. 2*l.*

MEDICIS. Unächter Acacien-Baum. 5 vols. in 9, 8vo. coloured plates. Leipsig, 1796-1798. 15*s.*

MEIDINGER. Icones Piscium Austriæ indigenorum in-fol. With 50 coloured plates. Viennæ, 1785-1794. 3*l.*

MEINICKE (CARL E.) Die Sudfeeuvölker und das Christenthum. 8vo. Brenslaw, 1844. 4*s.*

MEISSNER. Die Kinderkrankheiten. 2 vols. 8vo. Leipsig, 1828. 15*s.*

MEMOIRES de la Société Géologique de France. *Deuxième séries,* tome premier. Première partie, avec 6 planches. Paris, 1844. 15*s.*

—— de l'Académie Impériale des Sciences de St. Pétersbourg. Tome V. année 1812. In-4. St. Pétersbourg, 1815. 15*s.*

—— de l'Académie des Sciences de Turin. 6 vol. in-4. Turin, 1784-1800. 3*l.*

—— de l'Académie Royal de Médecine de Paris. Tomes I. à X. Paris, 1828-43. Prix de chaque vol. 1*l.*

Les 10 vols. pris ensemble, 8l. 10s.

—— (nouveaux) de l'Académie Royale des Sciences et Belles-Lettres, 1772-73. 2 vol. in-4. Berlin. 1*l.* 10*s.*

—— de la Société de Physique et d'Histoire Naturelle de Genève. Vol. VII. Part II. In-4. Genève, 1836. 10*s.*

—— de la Société Médicale d'observations. 2 vol. In-8. Paris, 1837-1843. 16*s.*

MENEGHINI. Richerche sulla Shuttura des Caule nelle Piante Monocotiledoni. 4to. with 10 plates. Padova, 1836. 16*s.*

MENONVILLE (THIERRY DE). Traité de la culture du Nopal, et de l'éducation de la Cochenille dans les colonies Françaises de l'Amérique. 2 vol. in-8. Paris. 6*s.*

MERZ (L.) Die neuren Verbesserungen am Microscope. 8vo. Müuchen, 1844. 2*s.* 6*d.*

MEYER (C. A.) Verzeichniss der Pflanzen, welche am westlichen Ufer des Caspischen Meeres gesammelt morden sind. 4to. St. Petersburg, 1831. 8*s.*

—— Novæ Plantarum Species. 4to. with plates. 3*s.*

—— (G. F. W.) Eine Anlage zur Flora des Königreichs Hannover. 2 vols. 8vo. with plates. Göttingen, 1822. 10*s.*

—— Chloris Hanoverana odor nach der natürlichten Familien geordnete Uebersicht den im Königreiche Hannover wildwachsenden sichtbar blühenden Gewächse und Farn. 4to. Göttingen, 1836. 1*l.*

—— Primitiæ Floræ Esqueboensis adjectis descriptionibus centum circiter stirpium novarum observationibusque criticis. 4to. with 2 plates. Göttingæ, 1818. 15*s.*

METCALFE (S.) The Natural History of Creation. In 1 vol. post 8vo. with plates. London, 1845.

(In the Press.)

MICHELIN. Iconographie zoophytologique description des polypiers fossiles de France. Liv. I. à XV. avec planches. 4to. Paris, 1843-44. Chaque, 3*s.*

MIKAN. Delectus Flora Fauna Brasiliensis. 4 fasc. fol. coloured plates. 1825. 6*l.*

MIQUEL (F. A. W.) Sertum Exoticum, contenant des Figures de Plantes Nouvelles, ou peu connues. Livraison I. 4to. with 5 plates and text. Rotterdam, 1843. 5*s.*

MIQUEL (F. A. W.) Commentarii Phytographiæ quibus varia rei Herbariæ capita, illustrator. Folio. Lugduni, 1840. 2*l.* 14*s.*

—— Systema Piperacearum. 2 vols. 8vo. Rotterdam, 1844. 1*l.* 2*s.*

MIRBEL (M.) Nouvelles recherches sur la structure et les développements de l'ovule végétale. In-4, with 10 plates. Paris, 1828. 5*s.*

MOHRENHEIM. Abhandlung über die Lutbindungskunst, mit kupfern 46. Large folio. Leipsig, 1803. 2*l.* 10*s.*

MONTE-BALDO. Descritta da Giovanni Pona Veronese, e due commenti, Marogna. 4to. plates. Venetia, 1617. 4*s.* 6*d.*

MOREAU. Icones Obstetricæ; a Series of 60 Plates, illustrative of the Art and Science of Midwifery in all its Branches. Edited, with Practical Remarks, by J. S. STREETER, M.R.C.S. Complete in 60 Plates, with Descriptions, in cloth boards, folio. London, 1841. Plain, 3*l.* 3*s.*; coloured, 6*l.* 6*s.*

—— (F. J.) Traité pratique des accouchemens. 2 vol. in-8, et atlas de 60 planches in-fol. Paris, 1838. 3*l.* Figs. col. 6*l.* 6*s.*

—— Le texte séparément, 2 vol. in-8, 14*s.*

MORITZI. Die Flora der Schweiz mit Besonderer Berücksichtigung ihrer Vertheilung nach Allgemein Physischen und Geologischen Momenten. 12mo. Zürich, 1844. 10*s.* 6*d.*

MORREN. Recherches sur la Rubéfaction des Eaux, et leur oxigénation par les animalcules et les algues. In-4, avec 7 pl. coloriées. 1841. 16*s.*

—— Responsio ad quæstionem ab ordine disciplinarum Mathematicarum, &c. 4to. with plates. 8*s.*

—— Recherches sur le mouvement et l'anatomie de stylidium graminifolium. 4to. plates. Bruxelles, 1838. 3*s.*

MORRISON. On the Distinction between Crime and Insanity; an Essay to which the Society for improving the Condition of the Insane awarded the Premium of Twenty Guineas. 8vo. London, 1844. 2*s.*

MORTON. Crania Americana; or, a Comparative View of the Skulls of various Aboriginal Nations of North and South America, to which is prefixed an Essay on the Varieties of the Human Species, illustrated by 78 plates, and a coloured map. Folio. Philadelphia, 1839. 6*l.*

MOSSLER'S Handbuch der Gewachskunde. Dritte anflage von H. G. L. REICHENBACH. 3 vols. 8vo. Altona, 1833. 1*l.* 4*s.*

MOXON (C.) An Introduction to Mineralogy; being the Natural System of Classification of Mineral and Metallic Bodies. 8vo. London, 1843. 9*s.*

MUHLFELD. Bemerkungen Berichtugungen und Zusatze zu illiger's Zusätzen. 8vo. Leipsig, 1812. 2*s.* 6*d.*

MULDER (C. J.) Uber den Werth und die Bedentung der Naturwissenchaften für die Medicin aus dem Hollandischen von Moleschott. 8vo. Heidelberg, 1844. 1*s.*

MULLER. Animalcula Infusoria, Fluviatilia, et Marina, quæ detexit, systematice descripsit, et ad vivum delineari curavit. Opus hoc posthumum, curâ FABRICII. 4to. with 50 plates. Haunlæ, 1786. 3*l.*

—— (J.) Albanien, Rumelien, und die österreichsmontenegrimische Gränze. 8vo. with a map. Prague, 1844. 4*s.* 6*d.*

—— Archiv für Anatomie und Physiologie. 8vo. mit Kupf. 1834-41. 1*l.* 4*s.* each year.

—— Handbuch der Physiologie des Menschen. 2 vols. 8vo. Coblentz, 1838-40. 2*l.*

—— Physiologie du Système Nerveux, ou recherches et expériences sur les diverses classes d'apparéils nerveux, les mouvemens, la voix, la parole, les sens et les facultés intellectuelles. Traduit de l'Allemand, par JOURDAN. 2 vols. in-8, avec fig. Paris, 1841. 16*s.*

—— Bau des Pentacrinus caput Medusæ. Folio, with 6 plates. Berlin, 1843. 12*s.*

—— Ueber die Compensation der Physischen Kräfte am Menschlichen Stimmorgan. 8vo. with 5 plates. Berlin, 1839. 4*s.*

MULLER (J.) Ueber den Glatten Hai des ARIS-
TOTELES und über die Verschiedenheiten unter
den Haifischenund Rochen in der Entwirk-
lung des Eies. Folio, with 6 plates. Berlin,
1842. 8*s.*
—— Ueber den feinern Bau und die formen
der Krankhaften Geschwülste. Folio, 4 Tafeln.
Berlin, 1838. 18*s.*
—— De glandularum secernentium structura pen-
itiori earumque prima Formatione in Homine at-
que Animalibus Commentatio Anatomica. Cum
Tabulis 16. Folio. Lipsiæ, 1830. 3*l.* 15*s.*
—— UND TROSCHEL. System der Asteriden.
4to. with 12 plates. Braunschweig, 1842.
1*l.* 16*s.*
—— (O.) Vermium Terrestrium et Fluviatilium,
seu Animalium, Infusorium, Helmintorum et
Testaceorum. 3 parts, 4to. Havniæ, 1773. 12*s.*
—— (O. F.) Hydrachnæ quas in Aquis Daniæ
Palustribus delexit et descripsit. 4to. with 11
plates. Leipsic, 1781. 10*s.*
—— (TH.) Synopsis Testaceorum. 8vo. Berolini,
1835. 6*s.*
MULSANT. Histoire naturelle des coléoptères
de France. 3 vols. in-8. Paris, 1844. 1*l.* 12*s.*
MUNSTER. Verzeichniss der in der Kreis-na-
turalien Sammlung zu Bayreuth Befindlichen
Petrefacten. 4to. with 22 plates. Leipzig,
1840. 2*l.*
MYLII. Memorabilium Saxoniæ Subterranæ.
4to. with 74 plates of Fossils. Leipsig, 1709. 5*s.*

NACCARI (F. L.) Flora Veneta. 6 vols. 4to. Ve-
nezia, 1826. 2*l.* 2*s.*
NEES AB ESENBECK. Sammlung schönblü-
hender gewächse. Text 4to. and atlas folio, with
100 col. pl. Dusseldorf, 1831. 5*l.*
—— Fraxinellæ, Plantarum Familia Naturalis.
With 11 folia plates. 5*s.*
—— Goethea Novum Plantarum Genus. 4to. with
3 folio plates. 2*s.* 6*d.*
—— De Polypore Pisacapani. 4to. with fol. pl. 2*s.* 6*d.*
—— Spiridens Movum Muscorum Diploperisto-
miorum Genus. 4to. with a coloured plate. 1*s.* 6*d.*
—— Fungi Javanici. 4to. with a col. pl. 3*s.*
—— Beschribung Officineller Pflanzen, texte seul.
1 vol. folio. Dusseldorf, 1829. 1*l.* 1*s.*
—— De Cinnamomo Disputatio, cum 7 tabulis ico-
nographicis. 4to. Bonn, 1823. 6*s.*
—— Genera Plantarum Floræ Germanicæ. 22 liv-
raisons, 8vo. containing 20 plates each, price per
livraison, 4*s.* Bonn, 1838-43.
—— Genera et Species Asterearum. 8vo. Vra-
tislaviæ, 1832. 7*s.* 6*d.*
—— Sammlung officineller pflanzen. 2 vols. ufol.
contenant 528 planches coloriées, and 1 vol. ufol.
de Texte. Dusseldorf, 1821-32. 15*l.* 15*s.*
—— UND WEIHE. Rubi Germanici. Folio. mit
52 planches. Elberfield, 1822-27. 4*l.*
NAGELII. Zeitschrift fur Wissenschaftliche Bo-
tanik. With 3 plates. Zurich, 1844. 7*s.*
NELATON. Elémens de pathologie chirurgicale.
Tome première. In-8. Paris, 1844. 8*s.*
NEUMANN C. G.) Pathologische untersuch als
Regulative des heilverfahrens. 2 vol. 8vo. Ber-
lin, 1841. 8*s.*
NICOLAI. Handbuch der gerichtlichen Medicin
nach dem gegenwärtigen Standpunkte dieser
Wissenschaft für Aerzte und Criminalisten. 8vo.
Berlin, 1841. 9*s.*
NOZEMAN UND SEPP. Nederlandsche Vogelen,
Volgens hunne huishoudlng, aert. en Eigens-
chappen Beschreeven. 5 vols. grand fol. avec
250 planches coloriées. Amsterdam, 1770-1829.
31*l.* 10*s.*

OBSERVATIONS sur l'histoire naturelle, sur la
physique, et sur la peinture, avec des planches
imprimées en couleur. 2 vol. in-4. Paris,
1752. 1*l.*
ŒDER ET MULLER. Flora Danica. 9 vols. fol.
coloured plates. Kopenhagen, 1766-92. 20*l.*
OKEN. Isis, Encyclopädische Zeitschrift vorzüg-
lich für Naturgeschichte, vergleichenden Anatomie und Physiologie. 30 vols. 4to. Leipzig,
1817-38. 38*l.*

OTTO ET PFEIFFER. Figures et Descriptions des
Cactées en Fleur. 5 livr. avec 70 planches, 4to.
col. Cassel, 1841-42. 1*l.*
OWEN (R.) Odontography, or a treatise on the
comparative Anatomy of the Teeth, their phy-
siological relations, mode of developement, and
Microscopic Structure in Vertebrate Animals.
  This splendid Work will be published in Three
Parts, each Part containing 50 Plates, with their
Description. When complete, it will form 1 vol.
of Letterpress, and an Atlas, royal 8vo. of 150
Plates, engraved by Mr. L. ALDOUS and Mr.
DINKEL. Parts I. and II. royal 8vo. 100 highly
engraved plates, with text, 1*l.* 11*s.* 6*d.* each.
  A few Copies are printed in 4to. and the Plates
Proofs on India Paper. 2*l.* 12*s.* 6*d.* each part.
*The Third and Last Part will be published in
January 1845.*

PALISOT (DE BEAUVOIS). Essai d'une nouvelle
agrostographie. 4to. avec 25 planches. Paris,
1812. 1*l.* 5*s.*
PALLAS. Miscellanea Zoologica. In-4, avec 14
pl. demie relié. Lugduni Batavorum, 1778. 1*l.*
—— Charakteristik die Thierpflanzen. Aus dem
Latein, übersetzt und mit Anmerkungen ver-
sehen von CHRIST. FRIEDR. WILKENS, und nach
seinem Tode herausg. von J. F. W. HERBST.
4to. Nürnberg, 1787. 18*s.*
PALSTERCAMP (A.) Théorie des Volcans.
3 vol. in-8, et atlas fol. Paris, 1835. 2*l.*
PANCOVII Herbarium portatile. 4to. avec 1362
gravures sur bois. Berlin, 1654. 4*s.*
PANDER. Entwickelungsgeschichte des Hühn-
chens im Eye. Fol. plates. Würzburg, 1817.
1*l.* 15*s.*
—— Historium metamorphoses quam ovum incu-
batum. 8vo. Worceburgi, 1817. 2*s.* 6*d.*
PANIZZA (B.) Annotazioni Chirurgiche sulla
Glandola parotide. 4to. with 2 plates. Milano,
1843. 4*s.*
PANZER. Fauna Insectorum, 1-140 fasc. illum.
18mo. Nürnberg, 1792-1838. 20*l.*
PARE (AMBROISE). Œuvres complètes, revues et
collationnées sur toutes les éditions, avec les
variantes; ornées de 217 planches et du portrait
de l'auteur, accompagnées de notes historiques et
critiques, et précédées d'une Introduction sur
l'origin et les progrès de la chirurgie en Occident
du VI.-XVI. siècle et sur la vie et les ouvrages
d'Ambroise Paré, par J. F. MALGAIGNE, chirur-
gien de l'hospice de Bicêtre, professeur agrégé à
la Faculté de Paris, &c. 3 vol. grand in-8 à deux
colonnes, avec un grand nombre de figures intercalées dans le texte. Paris, 1841. 1*l.* 16*s.*
PARENT-DUCHATELET. De la Prostitution
dans la ville de Paris, considérée sous les rapports de l'hygiène publique, de la morale et de
l'administration, ouvrage appuyé de documens
statistiques puisés dans les Archives de la Pré-
fecture de Police, avec cartes et tableaux. Seconde édition revue et corrigée, ornée du portrait de l'auteur gravé. 2 forts vol. in-8. Paris,
1837. 16*s.*
—— Hygiène publique, ou Mémoire sur les ques-
tions les plus importantes de l'hygiène appliquée
aux professions et aux travaux d'utilité publique.
2 forts vol. in-8, avec 18 pl. Paris, 1836. 16*s.*
PASSOT. Barème du vendeur et de l'acheteur
en poids décimaux et mesures métriques. 4to.
Paris, 1840. 4*s.* 6*d.*
PAYEN. Mémoires sur les développements des
végétaux. 4to. avec 16 planches. Paris, 1844.
1*l.* 4*s.*
PAYKULL. Fauna Suecica Insecta. 3 vols. 8vo.
Upsaliæ, 1800. 1*l.* 4*s.*
PELLETIER. A fine Portrait of. Folio. 3*s.* 6*d.*
PERSOON. Icones Pictæ Rariorum Fungorum.
4to. with 18 coloured plates. Paris, 1805. 1*l.* 5*s.*
—— Synopsis Plantarum, seu Enchiridium Bo-
tanicum. 2 vols. 12mo. Parisiis, 1807. 18*s.* 6*d.*
—— Mycologia Europæa. 3 vols. in-8, avec col.
pl. Erlangæ, 1828. 2*l.* 10*s.*
—— Icones et Descriptiones Fungorum minus cog-
nitorum. 4to. avec 14 planches coloriées. Leip-
sig, no date. 15*s.*

PETTER. Botanischer Wegweiser in der gegend von spalate. 18mo. Zaræ, 1832. 3s.

PHARMACEUTISCHES Central-Blatt für 1830, 32, 33, 34, 35, 36, 37, 38, 39, 40. In cloth boards. Leipzig. Each year, 15s.

PHARMACOPÉE FRANCAISE, ou code des médicamens; ou nouvelle traduction du codex medicamentarius, sive pharmacopœa Gallica, par F. S. RATIER, augmentée de notes et un appendice, contenant la formule et la mode de préparation des nouveaux médicamens, dont la pratique s'est enrichie jusqu'à nos jours, par O. HENRY. 1 vol. in-8. Paris, 1827. 8s.

PHILIPP. Zur Diagnostik der Lungen und herzkrankheiten Physicalischen Zeichen der Auscultation und Percussion. 8vo. fig. Berlin, 1836. 6s.

PHILIPPI Enumeratio Molluscorum Siciliæ. 12 planches. 4to. Berolini, 1836. 1l. 8s.
—— Vol. II. 4to. plates. Halle, 1844. 1l. 12s.

PICOT (DE LA PEIROUSE). Description de plusieurs nouvelles espèces d'orthocératites et d'ostracites, avec 13 planches. Folio. Erlang, 1781. 1l. 8s.
—— Figures de la Flore des Pyrénées avec les Descriptions. Folio, avec 11 planches coloriées. Paris, 1795. 10s.

PIDDINGTON. An English Index to the Plants of India. 8vo. Calcutta, 1832. 4s. 6d.

PIERER. Universal Lexicon oder Encyclopadische Wörterbuch. 26 vols. 8vo. half-bound. Altenburg, 1838-36. 9l.

PINEL. Traité de Pathologie du Cerveau. 8vo. Paris, 1844. 7s.

PITARO. La Science de la Sétifère, ou l'art de produire la sole avec avantage et sûreté, avec 7 planches. 8vo. Paris, 1828. 7s.

PLUMIER. Descriptions des plantes de l'Amérique, avec 108 planches fol. Paris. 1l. 10s.

POHL. Tentamen floræ Bohemiæ. 2 vols. 8vo. in 1. Prague, 1810-1815. 8s.

POILROUX. Médecine Légale criminelle Manuel à l'usage des médecins de toutes les classes des étudiens en médecine et des magistrats. 8vo. Paris, 1837. 7s.

POIRET (l'Abbé). Voyage en Barbarie, ou lettres écrites de l'ancienne Numidie en 1785 et 1786. 2 vol. in-8. Paris, 1789. 6s.

POISSON. A fine Portrait of. Folio. 5s.

POLANSKY (E.) Grundrisz zu einer Lehre von den Ohren-Krankheiten. 8vo. Wien, 1842. 4s.

POLLICH. Historia Plantarum in Palatinat-Electorali, sponte Nascentium incepta. 3 vols. 8vo. Mannheim, 1777. 12s. 6d.

POPPE. Ausführliche Volks-Gewerlslehre oder Allgemeine und befondere Technologie. 8vo. Stuttg. 15s.

POUILLET. Elémens de physiques expérimentale et de météorologie. Quatrième édition. 2 vol. in-8. Paris, 1845. 18s.

PREISS. Enumeratio Plantarum quas in Australasia Occidentali et Meridionali-occidentali, annis 1838-41. 8vo. Hamburgi. 8s.
—— (B.) Die neuere Physiologie in ihrem Einfiusse auf die nähere Kenntnis des Pfortadersystems in gesunden und kranken Fustande. 8vo. Breslau 1844. 4s.

PRICHARD. The Natural History of Man; comprising Inquiries into the Modifying Influences of Physical and Moral Agencies on the different Tribes of the Human Family. Illustrated with 44 coloured and 5 plain plates, engraved on steel, and 97 woodcuts. 1 vol. royal 8vo. elegantly bound in cloth. London, 1845. 1l. 13s. 6d. *Second edition, enlarged.*
—— Appendix to the First Edition of the Natural History of Man. Consisting of 4 sheets of text, and 6 coloured plates. 8vo. London, 1845. 3s. 6d.
—— Researches into the Physical History of Mankind. *Third Edition.* 4 vol. 8vo. London, 1841-44. 3l. 4s.
—— Illustrations to the Researches into the Physical History of Mankind. *Atlas of 44 coloured and 5 plain plates engraved on steel.* 1 vol. 8vo. London, 1844. 18s.

PRICHARD. Six Ethnographical Maps, large folio, coloured, with a sheet of letterpress, in illustration and as a complement of his works, "The Natural History of Man," and "Researches into the Physical History of Mankind." London, 1845. 1l. 1s. In cloth boards, 1l. 4s.
—— On the Different Forms of Insanity, in relation to Jurisprudence. Dedicated, by permission, to the Right Honourable LORD LYNDHURST, Chancellor of England. In 1 vol. post 8vo. London, 1842. 8s.

PRONY (M. de). Leçons de Mécanique Analytique, données à l'école impériale polytechnique. 2 vols. 4to. Paris, 1810.

PURKINJE (A. Y.) De cellulis antherarum fibrosis nec non De Granorum Pollinarum formis Commentatio Phytotomica. 4to. with 18 plates. Vratislaviæ, 1830. 12s.

QUETELET sur l'homme et le développement de ses facultés, ou essai de physique sociale. 2 vol. in-12. Bruxelles, 1836. 7s.

RABENHORST. Deutschlands Kryptogamen-Flora oder Handbuch zur Bestimmung der Kryptogamischen Gewächse Deutschlands der Schweiz, des Lombardisch-Benetianischen Konigreichs und Istreins. Vol. I. 8vo. Leipzig, 1844. 14s.

RACIBORSKI (M. A.) De la Puberté et de l'age critique chez la femme. In-12. Paris, 1844. 6s.

RAIMANN, Handbuch der Speciellen Medicinische und Thérapie. 2 vol. in-8. Wien, 1839. 1l. 4s.

RAMON (DE LA SAGRA.) Histoire physique, politique, et naturelle, de l'Ile de Cuba. 51 livraisons, fol. coloured plates. Paris, 1840-44. Price of each part, 12s. 6d.

RASPAIL (F. V.) Histoire naturelle de la santé et de la maladie chez les végétaux et chez les animaux en générale, et en particulier chez l'homme. 2 vol. in-8, avec planches. Paris, 1843. 1l. 4s.
—— Nouveau système de chimie organique, fondé sur de nouvelles méthodes d'observations, précédé d'un traité complet sur l'art d'observer et de manipuler en grand et en petit dans le laboratoire et sur le port-objet du microscrope. Deuxième édition, entièrement refondue, accompagné d'un atlas in-4 de 20 planches de figures dessinées d'après nature, gravées et coloriées avec le plus grand soin. 3 vol. in-8, atlas in-4. Paris, 1838. 1l. 10s.
—— Nouveau système de physiologie végétale et de botanique. 2 vol. in-8, et atlas de planches. Paris, 1837. 1l. 10s. Col. 2l. 10s.

RATIER. Pharmacopée Française, ou code des médicamens, nouvelle traduction du Codex Medicamentarius, sive Pharmacopœia Gallica. In-8. Paris, 1827. 8s.
—— Lettre sur la Syphilis. In-8. Paris, 1844. 1s. 6d.

RATZEBURG (J. T. C.) Die Forst-Insecten. 3 vols. 4to. with 37 plates. Berlin, 1837. 3l. 3s.
—— Entomologische Beiträge. 4to. 5s.
—— Animadversiones quædam ad peloiarum indolem definiendam spectantes. 4to. with a plate. Berolini. 8s.

RAU. Die Entzündung der Regenbogenhaut. 8vo. Bern-und-St. Gallen, 1844. 6s.

RAYER. A Theoretical and Practical Treatise on the Diseases of the Skin. Translated by R. WILLIS, M.D. Second edition, remodelled and enlarged, in 1 thick vol. 8vo. of 1300 pages, with atlas royal 4to. of 26 plates, finely engraved and coloured with the greatest care, exhibiting 400 Varieties of Cutaneous Affections. 4l. 8s. London, 1835. The Text separately, 8vo. in boards, 1l. 8s. The Atlas 4to. separately, in boards, 3l. 10s.
See WILLIS.
—— Traité des maladies des reins et des altérations de la sécrétion urinaire, étudiés en elles-mêmes et dans leurs rapports; avec les maladies des urétères, de la vessie, et la prostate, de l'urètre, &c. 3 forts vol. in-8. Paris, 1839-41. 1l. 4s.

RAYER (P.) Traité théorique et pratique des maladies de la peau. Deuxième édition, entièrement refondue. 3 forts vol. in-8, accompagnés d'un bel atlas de 26 planches, in grand-4, gravées et coloriées avec les plus grand soin, représentant en 400 figures les différentes maladies de la peau et leurs variétés. Paris, 1835. Prix de texte seul, 1l. 3s.
—— Prix de l'ouvrage complet, 3 vol. in-8 et atlas in-4 cart. 4l. 8s.
—— Prix de l'atlas seul, avec explication raisonnée, grand in-4 cart, 3l. 10s.
—— Le bel atlas pour cet ouvrage, représentant les diverses altérations morbides des reins, de la vessie, de la prostate, des urétères, de l'urètre, a été publié en 12 livraisons contenant chacune 5 planches grand in-folio, gravées et magnifiquement coloriées d'après nature, avec un texte descriptif. Ce bel ouvrage, composé de 60 planches grand in-folio, est complet. Paris, 1841. 9l. 12s.
RECEUIL de médecine vétérinaire. Première année. Tome I. in-8. Paris, 1824. 12s.
REGENFUSS (F. M.) Auserlesene Schnelkenmuscheln und andere Schaalthiere. Folio, with 12 col. pl. Kopenhagen, 1758. 6l. 6s.
REICHENBACH. Flora Germanica. 3 vols. 18mo. Lipsiæ, 1830. 1l.
—— Allgemeine Pflanzenkunde. 4to. with 8 coloured plates. Leipzig, 1838. 6s.
—— Handbuch des Natürlichen Pflanzensystems, nach allen feinen Classen, Ordnungen und Familien. 8vo. Dresden, 1837. 1l.
—— Floræ Lipsiensis Pharmaceuticæ Specimen. Lipsiæ. 2s.
—— Die Tand Süfrwasser und see Conchilien, mit 68 tafmehr, 800 abbeldungen enthaltend. Royal 8vo. half-boards. Leipzig, 1842. 1l. 16s.
REICHOLDT u. REIDER. Die Pharmaceutische Waarenkunde und Waarenbereitung. 8vo. Leipzig, 1844. 6s.
REIL. Archiv für die Physiologie. 12 vols. bound. Halle, 1795-1815. 5l.
REQUIN. Elémens de pathologie médicale. Vol. I. in-8. Paris, 1843. 7s.
RETZII Observationes Botanicæ sex fasciculis comprehensæ. Cum 19 pl. fol. col. Lipsiæ, 1791. 1l.
REUSS (A. E.) Geognotische Skizzen aus Böhmen. 2 vols. 8vo. with plates. Prague, 1844. 12s.
RHÆDE et CASEARIUM. Hortus Indicus Malabaricus continens Regni Malabarici apud Indos Celeberrimi omnis Generis Plantas rariores. 2 vols. folio, with numerous plates. Amsterdam, 1668. 15s.
RICARD (J. A.) Physiologie et hygiène du magnétiseur; régime diététique du magnétisé, &c. In-12. Paris, 1844. 3s. 6d.
RICHARDSON (G. F.) Geology for Beginners, comprising a Familiar Exposition of the Elements of Geology and its Associate Sciences, Mineralogy, Fossil Conchology, Fossil Botany, and Palæontology. 1 vol. post 8vo. illustrated by 251 Woodcuts. Second edition. 1843. 10s. 6d.
RICHTERN. Saxoniæ Electoralis Miraculosa Terra. 4to. 61 plates. 1732. 5s.
RICORD (Ph.) Traité pratique des maladies vénériennes, ou recherches critiques et expérimentales sur l'inoculation appliquée à l'étude de ces maladies, suivies d'un résumé thérapeutique et d'un formulaire spécial. In-8. Paris, 1838. 9s.
—— Atlas des maladies vénériennes. 7 livraisons, 4to. chaque contenant 4 planches coloriées. 2l. 2s. L'ouvrage sera complet en 20 livraisons.
RIDINGER. A Collection of 38 splendid Engravings of Animals, *Mammalia.* Folio. 19s.
—— Of Birds. 4 plates, folio. 3s.
RIEM. Oekonomisch-Veterinärisches Unterricht über die Zucht, Wartung und Stallung der Pferde. 7 parts, 4to. with plates, bound in 1 vol. Leipzig, 1799-1802. 1l. 15s.
RILLIET et BARTHEZ. Traité clinique et pratique des maladies des enfans. 3 vol. in-8. Paris, 1843. 1l. 1s.
ROEHMANN (L.) Handbuch der Topographischen Anatomie. 12mo. Leipzig, 1844. 16s.

RIECKE (V. A.) Die Neuern Arzneimittel ihre physischen und chemischen Eigenschaften Bereitungsweisen, Wirkungen auf den Gesunden und Kranken Organismus und Therapeutische Benutzung. 8vo. Stuttgart, 1840. 12s. *Second edition.*
ROCHE, SANSON, et LENOIR. Nouveaux élémens de pathologie médico-chirurgicale, ou traité théorique et pratique de médecine et de chirurgie. Quatrième édition considérablement augmentée. 5 forts vol. in-8. Paris, 1844. 1l. 16s.
ROEDERER. Elémens de l'Art des Accouchemens, augmentés des observations sur les accouchemens laborieux, avec figures. 8vo. Paris, 1765. 5s.
ROGNETTA. Traité philosophique et clinique d'Ophthalmologie, basé sur les principes de la Thérapeutique Dynamique. 8vo. Paris, 1844. 9s.
ROODS (H. C.) Spinal Affections. A popular Lecture on Disorders and Diseases of the Spine, in which the Causes, Nature, Symptoms, and Curative Treatment of these Affections, are investigated and explained. 12mo. with 2 woodcuts. London, 1841. 2s.
ROSE. Traité pratique d'analyse chimique, suivie de tables servant dans les analyses àcalculer à la quantité d'une substance d'après celle qui a été trouvée dans une autre substance; trad. de l'Allemand sur la quatrième édition, par A. J. L. Jourdan. Nouvelle édition avec des additions, par Peligot. 2 vol. in-8, fig. Paris, 1843. 16s.
ROSENBAUM. Zur Geschichteund Kritik der Lehre vonden Hautkrankheiten. 8vo. Halle, 1844. 4s.
ROSER (W.) Handbuch der anatomischen Chirurgie. 8vo. Tübingen, 1844. 12s.
ROSES (les), Paintes par P. J. Redoute, décrites et classées selon leur ordre naturel par C. A. Thory. Troisième édition. 3 vols. gr. in-8, avec fig. col. Paris, 1828. 10l.
ROTH. Novæ Plantarum species præsertin Indiæ Orientalis, ex collectione Doct. Benj. Heyne. 8vo. Halber-stadii, 1821. 5s.
ROTHII (A. G.) Catalecta Botanica, quibus plantæ novæ et minus cognitæ describuntur et illustrantur. 3 vols. 8vo. Mit illum. tafeln. Leipzig, 1806. 1l.
ROTTBOLL. Descriptionum et Iconum rariores et pro maxima parte. Novas plantas illustrat. Fol. avec 21 planches. Hafniæ, 1773. 15s.
ROYEN. Flora Leydensia, prodromus exhibens plantas quæ in Horto Academico Lugduno-Batavo abundantur. 8vo. 1740. 3s. 6d.
RUDOLPHI Entozoorum Synopsis. Cum 3 Tabulis. 8vo. Berlin, 1819. 1l.
—— Entozoorum sive vermium intestinalium. 3 vols. 8vo. Amsterdam, 1808. 1l. 15s.
—— Dissertatio anatomica de oculi quibusdam partibus. 4to. Gryphiæ. 3s.
—— Grundriss der Physiologie. 2 vols. in 1, 8vo. bd. Berlin, 1821. 15s.
RUNGE. Einleitung in die Technische Chimie für Jederman. Mit 150 in text Befundlichen Tafeln. 8vo. Berlin, 1836. 18s.
RUPPEL (E. Dr.) Atlas zu der Reise in Nördlichen Afrika. Vol. I. containing 120 plates, coloured and plain, folio. Vol. II. Neue Wirbelthiere zu der Fauna von Abyssinien gehörig, containing 94 plates, coloured and plain, folio. Franckfurt, 1826-40. 21l.
RUST. Helkologie, oder Lehre von den Geschwären. 4to. mit 12 illum. Kupf. Berlin, 1842. 3l.

—— (Dr. C.) De ulcerum diagnosi et aetiologia Nonnulla. 4to. with 7 plates coloured, in folio. Bertolini, 1831. 8s.
RYAN (M.) The Philosophy of Marriage, in its Social, Moral, and Physical Relations; with an Account of the Diseases of the Genito-Urinary Organs, with the physiology of Generation in the Vegetable and Animal Kingdoms. Fourth edition, very much improved. 1 vol. 12mo. London, 1843. 6s.

CPSIA information can be obtained at www.ICGtesting.com
Printed in the USA
LVOW052141140113

315671LV00025B/1967/P